UNDERGROUND
CLINICAL VIGNETTES

··

INTERNAL MEDICINE VOL. I

Classic Clinical Cases for
USMLE Step 2 Review [56 cases]

VIKAS BHUSHAN, MD
University of California, San Francisco, Class of 1991
Series Editor, Diagnostic Radiologist

TAO LE, MD
University of California, San Francisco, Class of 1996
Yale-New Haven Hospital, Resident in Internal Medicine

CHIRAG AMIN, MD
University of Miami, Class of 1996
Orlando Regional Medical Center, Resident in Orthopaedic Surgery

HOANG NGUYEN
Northwestern University, Class of 2000

VISHAL PALL, MBBS
Government Medical College, Chandigarh, India, Class of 1996

DIEGO RUIZ
University of California, San Francisco, Class of 1999

©1999 by S2S Medical Publishing

DISTRIBUTED by Blackwell Science, Inc.
Editorial Office:
Commerce Place, 350 Main Street, Malden, Massachusetts 02148, USA

DISTRIBUTORS

USA

Commerce Place
350 Main Street
Malden, Massachusetts 02148
(Telephone orders: 800-215-1000 or
781-388-8250;
fax orders: 781-388-8270)

Canada

Login Brothers Book Company
324 Saulteaux Crescent
Winnipeg, Manitoba, R3J 3T2
(Telephone orders: 204-224-4068;
Telephone: 800-665-1148;
fax: 800-665-0103

Australia

Blackwell Science Pty Ltd.
54 University Street
Carlton, Victoria 3053
(Telephone orders: 03-9347-0300;
fax orders: 03-9349-3016)

Outside North America and Australia

Blackwell Science, Ltd.
c/o Marston Book Service, Ltd.
P.O. Box 269
Abingdon
Oxon OX14 4YN
England
(Telephone orders: 44-01235-465500;
fax orders: 44-01235-465555)

ISBN: 1-890061-20-4
TITLE: Underground Clinical Vignettes: Internal Medicine, Vol. I

Editor: Andrea Fellows
Typesetter: Vikas Bhushan using MS Word97
Printed and bound by Capital City Press

Printed in the United States of America
99 00 01 02 6 5 4 3 2

Contributors

. . . .

JOSE M. FIERRO, MD
Brookdale Hospital, Resident in Medicine/Pediatrics

JOSEPH LIM
Northwestern University, Class of 1999

RACHAN REDDY
Northwestern University, Class of 1999

RAJIV ROY
USC School of Medicine, Class of 1999

JOHN SCHILLING
University of Chicago, Class of 1999

ERIC TAYLOR
UCLA School of Medicine, Class of 1999

ASHRAF ZAMAN, MBBS
International Medical Graduate

Faculty Reviewers

. . . .

CHRISTOPHER COSGROVE, MD
Yale University School of Medicine, Chief Resident in Internal Medicine

EUNICE WANG, MD
Yale University School of Medicine, Resident in Internal Medicine

Acknowledgments

Throughout the production of this book, we have had the support of many friends and colleagues. Special thanks to our business manager, Gianni Le Nguyen. For expert computer support, Tarun Mathur and Alex Grimm. For additional copy editing services, Erica Simmons. For design suggestions, Sonia Santos and Elizabeth Sanders.

For authorship, editing, proofreading, and assistance across the vignette series, we collectively thank Chris Aiken, Kris Alden, Ted Amanios, Henry Aryan, Natalie Barteneva, MD, Adam Bennett, Ross Berkeley, MD, Archana Bindra, MBBS, Sanjay Bindra, MBBS, Aminah Bliss, Tamara Callahan, MD, MPP, Aaron Caughey, MD, MPP, Deanna Chin, Vladimir Coric, MD, Vladimir Coric, Sr., MD, Ronald Cowan, MD, PhD, Ryan Crowley, Daniel Cruz, Zubin Damania, Rama Dandamudi, MD, Sunit Das, Brian Doran, MD, Alea Eusebio, Thomas Farquhar, Jose Fierro, MBBS, Tony George, MD, Parul Goyal, Sundar Jayaraman, Eve Kaiyala, Sudhir Kakarla, Seth Karp, MD, Bertram Katzung, MD, PhD, Aaron Kesselheim, Jeff Knake, Sharon Kreijci, Christopher Kosgrove, MD, Warren Levinson, MD, PhD, Eric Ley, Joseph Lim, Andy Lin, Daniel Lee, Scott Lee, Samir Mehta, Gil Melmed, Michael Murphy, MD, MPH, Dan Neagu, MD, Deanna Nobleza, Craig Nodurft, Henry Nguyen, Linh Nguyen, MD, Vishal Pall, MBBS, Paul Pamphrus, MD, Thao Pham, MD, Michelle Pinto, Riva Rahl, Aashita Randeria, Rachan Reddy, Rajiv Roy, Diego Ruiz, Sanjay Sahgal, MD, Mustafa Saifee, MD, Louis Sanfillipo, MD, John Schilling, Sonal Shah, Nutan Sharma, MD, PhD, Andrew Shpall, Kristy Smith, Tanya Smith, Vipal Soni, Brad Spellberg, Merita Tan, MD, Eric Taylor, Jennifer Ty, Anne Vu, MD, Eunice Wang, MD, Lynna Wang, Andy Weiss, Thomas Yoo, and Ashraf Zaman, MBBS. Please let us know if your name has been missed or misspelled and we will be happy to make the change in the next edition.

For generously contributing images to the entire *Underground Clinical Vignette* Step 2 series, we collectively thank the staff at Blackwell Science in Oxford, Boston, and Berlin as well as:

- Alfred Cuschieri, Thomas P.J. Hennessy, Roger M. Greenhalgh, David I. Rowley, Pierce A. Grace (*Clinical Surgery*, © 1996 Blackwell Science), Figures 13.23, 13.35b, 13.51, 15.13, 15.2.

- John Axford (*Medicine*, © 1996 Blackwell Science), Figures f 3.10, 2.103a, 2.110b, 3.20a, 3.20b, 3.25b, 3.38a, 5.9Bi, 5.9Bii, 6.41a, 6.41b, 6.74b, 6.74c, 7.78ai, 7.78aii, 7.78b, 8.47b, 9.9e, f 3.17, f 3.36, f 3.37, f 5.27, f 5.28, f 5.45a, f 5.48, f 5.49a, f 5.50, f 5.65a, f 5.67, f 5.68, f 8.27a, AX10.120b, 11.63b, 11.63c, 11.68a, 11.68b, 11.68c, 12.37a, 12.37b.

Table of Contents

Preface

....

This series was developed to address the nearly universal presence of clinical vignette questions on the USMLE Step 2. It is designed to supplement and complement *First Aid for the USMLE Step 2* (Appleton & Lange). Bidirectional cross-linking to appropriate High-Yield Facts in the second edition of *First Aid for the USMLE Step 2* has been implemented.

Each book uses a series of approximately 50 "**supra-prototypical**" **cases as a way to condense testable facts and associations.** The clinical vignettes in this series are designed to incorporate as many testable facts as possible into a cohesive and memorable clinical picture. The vignettes represent composites drawn from general and specialty textbooks, reference books, thousands of USMLE-style questions and the personal experience of the authors and reviewers. Additionally, we present "Associated Diseases" as a way to teach the most critical facts about a larger number of diseases that do not justify an entire case. **The "Associated Diseases" list is NOT complete and does not represent differential diagnoses.**

Although each case tends to present all the signs, symptoms, and diagnostic findings for a particular illness, **patients generally will not present with such a "complete" picture either clinically or on the Step 2 exam.** Cases are not meant to simulate a potential real patient or an exam vignette. All the **boldfaced "buzzwords" are for learning purposes** and are not necessarily expected to be found in any one patient with the disease. **Similarly, the images for each case are for learning purposes only, were derived from a variety of textbooks, and may not match the clinical vignette in all respects.** Images are labeled [A]–[D] and represent 1–4 images of varying sizes, with locations corresponding to a left-to-right, top-to-bottom lettering system.

Definitions of selected important terms are placed within the vignettes in (= SMALL CAPS) in parentheses. Other parenthetical remarks often refer to the pathophysiology or mechanism of disease. The format should also help students learn to present cases succinctly during oral "bullet" presentations on clinical rotations. The cases are meant to be read as a condensed review, not as a primary reference.

The information provided in this book has been prepared with a great deal of thought and careful research. This book should not, however, be considered your sole source of information. Corrections, suggestions, and submissions of new cases are encouraged and will be acknowledged and incorporated in future editions.

Abbreviations

. . . .

5-ASA - 5-aminosalicylic acid
ABGs - arterial blood gases
ABVD - adriamycin/bleomycin/vincristine/dacarbazine
ACE - angiotensin-converting enzyme
ACTH - adrenocorticotropic hormone
ADH - antidiuretic hormone
AI - aortic insufficiency
AIDS - acquired immunodeficiency syndrome
ALL - acute lymphocytic leukemia
ALT - alanine transaminase
AML - acute myelogenous leukemia
ANA - antinuclear antibody
ARDS - adult respiratory distress syndrome
ASD - atrial septal defect
ASO - anti-streptolysin O
AST - aspartate transaminase
AV - arteriovenous
BE - barium enema
BP - blood pressure
BUN - blood urea nitrogen
CAD - coronary artery disease
CALLA - common acute lymphoblastic leukemia antigen
CBC - complete blood count
CHF - congestive heart failure
CK - creatine kinase
CLL - chronic lymphocytic leukemia
CML - chronic myelogenous leukemia
CMV - cytomegalovirus
CNS - central nervous system
COPD - chronic obstructive pulmonary disease
CPK - creatine phosphokinase
CSF - cerebrospinal fluid
CT - computed tomography
CVA - cerebrovascular accident
CXR - chest x-ray
DIC - disseminated intravascular coagulation
DKA - diabetic ketoacidosis
DM - diabetes mellitus
DTRs - deep tendon reflexes
DVT - deep venous thrombosis
EBV - Epstein–Barr virus
ECG - electrocardiography
Echo - echocardiography
EF - ejection fraction
EGD - esophagogastroduodenoscopy
EMG - electromyography
ERCP - endoscopic retrograde cholangiopancreatography
ESR - erythrocyte sedimentation rate
FEV - forced expiratory volume

Abbreviations - continued

FNA - fine needle aspiration
FTA-ABS - fluorescent treponemal antibody absorption
FVC - forced vital capacity
GFR - glomerular filtration rate
GH - growth hormone
GI - gastrointestinal
GU - genitourinary
HAV - hepatitis A virus
HEENT - head, eyes, ears, nose, and throat
HIV - human immunodeficiency virus
HLA - human leukocyte antigen
HPI - history of present illness
HR - heart rate
HS - hereditary spherocytosis
ID/CC - identification and chief complaint
IDDM - insulin-dependent diabetes mellitus
Ig - immunoglobulin
IM - intramuscular
JVP - jugular venous pressure
KUB - kidneys/ureter/bladder
LDH - lactate dehydrogenase
LES - lower esophageal sphincter
LFTs - liver function tests
LP - lumbar puncture
LV - left ventricular
LVH - left ventricular hypertrophy
Lytes - electrolytes
MCHC - mean corpuscular hemoglobin concentration
MCV - mean corpuscular volume
MEN - multiple endocrine neoplasia
MGUS - monoclonal gammopathy of undetermined significance
MHC - major histocompatibility complex
MI - myocardial infarction
MOPP - mechlorethamine/vincristine (Oncovorin)/procarbazine/prednisone
MR - magnetic resonance (imaging)
NHL - non-Hodgkin's lymphoma
NIDDM - non-insulin-dependent diabetes mellitus
NPO - nil per os (nothing by mouth)
NSAID - nonsteroidal anti-inflammatory drug
PA - posteroanterior
PBS - peripheral blood smear
PE - physical exam
PFTs - pulmonary function tests
PMI - point of maximal intensity
PMN - polymorphonuclear leukocyte
PT - prothrombin time
PTCA - percutaneous transluminal angioplasty
PTH - parathyroid hormone
PTT - partial thromboplastin time

Abbreviations - continued

PUD - peptic ulcer disease
RBC - red blood cell
RPR - rapid plasma reagin
RR - respiratory rate
RS - Reed–Sternberg (cell)
RV - right ventricular
RVH - right ventricular hypertrophy
SBFT - small bowel follow-through
SIADH - syndrome of inappropriate secretion of ADH
SLE - systemic lupus erythematosus
STD - sexually transmitted disease
TFTs - thyroid function tests
tPA - tissue plasminogen activator
TSH - thyroid-stimulating hormone
TIBC - total iron-binding capacity
TIPS - transjugular intrahepatic portosystemic shunt
TPO - thyroid peroxidase
TSH - thyroid-stimulating hormone
TTP - thrombotic thrombocytopenic purpura
UA - urinalysis
UGI - upper GI
US - ultrasound
VDRL - Venereal Disease Research Laboratory
VS - vital signs
VT - ventricular tachycardia
WBC - white blood cell
WPW - Wolff–Parkinson–White (syndrome)
XR - x-ray

ID/CC	A 34-year-old **male** experiences an episode of **fainting** (= SYNCOPE) while cleaning the house.
HPI	Within the past six months, he has felt increasing **fatigue, palpitations,** and occasional **shortness of breath** (= DYSPNEA).
PE	VS: tachycardia (HR 122); **wide pulse pressure** (BP 140/50). PE: tall (190 cm) with long, thin limbs and high-arched palate; dislocated lens (= ECTOPIA LENTIS) in left eye (signs of Marfan's syndrome); **bobbing movement of head** (= DE MUSSET'S SIGN); crackles bilaterally at lung bases; **displaced PMI** (ventricular dilatation); S3 over apex; **high-pitched, decrescendo, blowing diastolic murmur** loudest at left sternal border; systolic blushing and diastolic blanching with gentle pressure on nail bed (= QUINCKE'S PULSE); **water-hammer pulse** (= CORRIGAN'S SIGN).
Labs	ECG: sinus rhythm with increased QRS amplitude and LVH.
Imaging	[A] CXR: LV enlargement (1) with cardiac apex displaced downward and to left; enlarged ascending aorta (2). Echo: LVH; aortic root dilatation; flutter of anterior leaflet; early closure of mitral valve.
Pathogenesis	Aortic insufficiency (= AORTIC REGURGITATION) may occur as a result of rheumatic heart disease (most common cause), infective endocarditis, Ehlers–Danlos syndrome, Marfan's syndrome with either proximal root dilatation or aortic root dissection (secondary to cystic medial necrosis), idiopathic aortic root dissection, syphilitic aortitis, or a congenital bicuspid valve. Aortic insufficiency leads to regurgitation of a fraction of the stroke volume back into the left ventricle during diastole, causing **increased LV filling pressure** and **end-diastolic volume,** which accounts for the **increased stroke volume and widened pulse pressure.** Ultimately, the increasing volume and filling pressure lead to CHF.
Epidemiology	Aortic insufficiency is a common valvular lesion that **occurs more frequently in males.** However, in cases with concomitant mitral valve disease, females predominate.

AORTIC INSUFFICIENCY

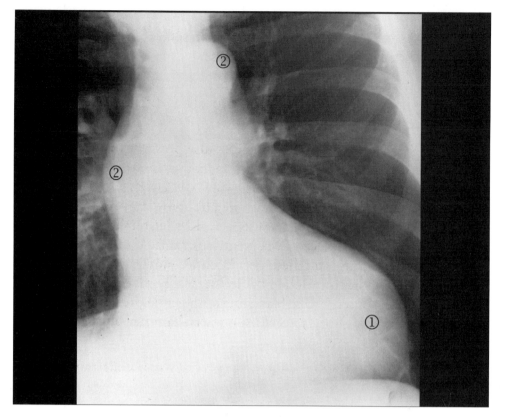

Management	Mild aortic insufficiency (AI) or asymptomatic severe AI with normal heart size with no evidence of LV systolic dysfunction requires only **bacterial endocarditis prophylaxis.** Symptomatic LV failure should be treated with digitalis, diuretics, and vasodilators. Patients with acute aortic insufficiency, medically refractory aortic insufficiency, increasing heart size, decreasing EF, or decompensated CHF require **aortic valve replacement.**
Complications	Untreated, AI eventually leads to **CHF;** patients are also at risk for developing **arrhythmias** and **infective endocarditis.**
Associated Diseases	◻ **Marfan's Syndrome** An autosomal-dominant defect in the fibrillin protein, which is required for collagen-fibril stability; presents with classic marfanoid features (tall, thin patients with long digits), cardiac valvular disease (mitral valve prolapse, mitral and aortic regurgitation), lenticular dislocation, and joint laxity; treatment is supportive; complications include cardiac disease.
	◻ **Syphilis** An STD caused by *Treponema pallidum* infection; divided into primary, secondary, tertiary, and

congenital; primary presents with a painless chancre in the genital area; secondary presents with a diffuse maculopapular rash, especially on the palms and soles, and with condylomata lata; tertiary presents with aortic aneurysms, gumma formation, and neurologic disease; congenital presents with fetal death or congenital abnormalities; screen with VDRL, RPR, or FTA-ABS (more specific) and darkfield microscopy; treat with penicillin.

AORTIC INSUFFICIENCY

ID/CC	A 39-year-old **male** complains of left-sided **chest pain at rest.**
HPI	The patient states that he has experienced increasing **fatigue** and a decrease in his normal activity. He adds that he has **shortness of breath with exertion.**
PE	VS: tachycardia; narrow pulse pressure. PE: **delayed, slow-rising carotid upstroke;** forceful apical beat **(LVH); soft S2** (secondary to diminished or absent aortic component); **harsh, late-peaking** (crescendo-decrescendo) **systolic ejection murmur** that is **loudest at right second intercostal space, radiating to carotids.**
Labs	ECG: LVH; ST depression and T-wave inversion.
Imaging	**[A]** CXR: poststenotic dilatation of the ascending aorta; other findings include LVH with calcification of the aortic valve. Echo: **bicuspid aortic valve;** left ventricle wall thickening; decreased valvular area.
Pathogenesis	Aortic stenosis may arise secondary to a congenital bicuspid aortic valve (60%), rheumatic valvular disease (10%), or idiopathic senile calcific aortic stenosis (common in the elderly). Obstruction to LV ejection leads to LV pressure overload and to a pressure gradient between the left ventricle and the aorta. In order to compensate for the increased wall stress, the left ventricle undergoes concentric hypertrophy, and patients usually progress from angina to syncope to CHF. Angina occurs as a result of increased oxygen demand coupled with decreased coronary artery perfusion; syncope occurs when the systemic venous resistance drops during exercise because the cardiac output cannot increase sufficiently, leading to hypotension and poor cerebral perfusion.
Epidemiology	Aortic stenosis is the **most common** cardiac valvular lesion; 80% of symptomatic adults are male.
Management	**Aortic valve replacement** for **symptomatic** patients and for **asymptomatic** patients with LVH and secondary ST-T changes on ECG. **Balloon valvuloplasty** may be used in infants, children, and young adults (whose valves are not calcified) and in adults who are poor surgical candidates; however, restenosis is common after nine months. **Pharmacologic therapy** has a limited role.

2.   AORTIC STENOSIS

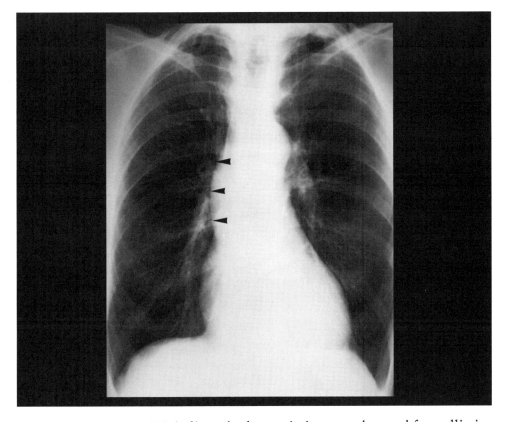

Digitalis and salt restriction may be used for palliation of CHF symptoms. Use diuretics cautiously. Patients should **avoid strenuous activity** and should receive **antibiotic prophylaxis** for all invasive medical and dental procedures.

Complications

Death may result from CHF or sudden cardiac death (presumably due to ventricular arrhythmias). Supraventricular arrhythmias, systemic emboli, and infective endocarditis may occur.

Associated Diseases

◻ **Aortic Sclerosis** Progressive calcification of a normal aortic valve in the elderly; presents with midsystolic murmur over the aorta; echo shows no narrowing of the valve area; no treatment is required.

◻ **Hypertrophic Cardiomyopathy** Ventricular outflow tract obstruction due to cardiac muscle hypertrophy; an autosomal-dominant inheritance pattern is seen in almost half of all cases; presents with dyspnea on exertion, angina, syncope, or sudden death (commonly associated with strenuous physical activity); ECG shows LVH; echo shows asymmetrical septal hypertrophy, systolic anterior motion of the mitral valve, and mitral regurgitation; treat with avoidance of competitive sports and strenuous physical activity, negative inotropic agents (beta-blockers and calcium channel blockers), amiodarone, possible surgical myomectomy of the interventricular septum.

◻ **Rheumatic Fever** Complication of group A streptococcal infection, secondary to autoantibodies directed against joints and heart valves; presents > 1 week after throat infection with migratory polyarthritis, endocarditis, and rash; antistreptococcal antibodies (e.g., ASO); treat with aspirin and penicillin; complications include permanent valvular disease.

AORTIC STENOSIS

ID/CC	A **39-year-old** male complains of recent-onset shortness of breath (= DYSPNEA), **fatigue,** and **decreased exercise tolerance.**
HPI	He states that the shortness of breath is **exacerbated when he stands and is relieved when he lies down.** He also states that he has developed **palpitations, malaise,** and **joint pains.** He has lost approximately 30 pounds in the past year.
PE	VS: **low-grade fever;** tachycardia; postural hypotension. PE: cachexia; clubbing; pallor; increased JVP; loud S1; **low-pitched sound in early diastole** (= "TUMOR PLOP" from myxoma stopping when it strikes the ventricular wall); Raynaud's phenomenon seen.
Labs	CBC: anemia; leukocytosis; thrombocytopenia. **ESR elevated;** hypergammaglobulinemia. ECG: sinus tachycardia.
Imaging	CXR: enlarged left atrium, pulmonary vascular redistribution, and RV enlargement. **[A]** Echo (schematic): single, mobile, **intracavitary,** pedunculated **mass in left atrium.**
Pathogenesis	Myxomas are true neoplasms that arise most commonly from the **left atrial septum** near the fossa ovalis; they are generally solitary, pedunculated, and 4–8 cm in length. These tumors frequently prolapse through the atrioventricular valve, yielding symptoms similar to **valvular stenosis.** However, they may also cause valvular trauma, leading to symptoms of **regurgitation.** In a small percentage of cases, the tumors are transmitted in an **autosomal-dominant** fashion. They may also arise as part of the NAME (= NEVI, ATRIAL MYXOMA, MYXOID NEUROFIBROMA, EPHELIDES) or LAMB (= LENTIGINES, ATRIAL MYXOMA, BLUE NEVI) syndromes.
Epidemiology	While the majority of tumors involving the heart are metastatic in origin, myxomas are the **most common primary cardiac tumor.** They exhibit no gender association, present most commonly between the third and sixth decades of life, and occur earlier when familial or associated with a syndrome.
Management	**Surgical excision;** screen first-degree relatives in young patients and those with multiple tumors.

ATRIAL MYXOMA

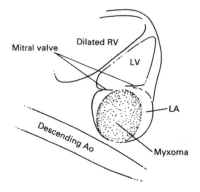

Complications	Metastatic **emboli**, infective endocarditis, and **syncope**.
Associated Diseases	◻ **Bacterial Endocarditis** Infection of prosthetic (usually with *S. epidermidis*), previously diseased (subacute IE, usually with *S. viridans*), or normal (acute IE, as in intravenous drug abusers, usually with *S. aureus*) heart valves; presents with fever, night sweats, and diffuse septic emboli (e.g., brain, kidney, liver, spleen); leukocytosis, elevated ESR, and positive blood cultures; echo reveals valvular vegetations; treat with 4–6 weeks of a penicillin or cephalosporin with or without aminoglycoside; complications include diffuse abscesses, valve destruction with resultant heart failure, sepsis, and multiple infarcts.

◻ **Mitral Stenosis** Fibrosis of the mitral valve commonly secondary to rheumatic heart disease; presents with dyspnea, hemoptysis, pulmonary edema, mid-diastolic rumble with opening snap at the apex, and RV heave; ECG shows P mitrale (due to left atrial enlargement), RVH, and right axis deviation; echo reveals calcification and stenosed valve orifice; treat with prophylaxis for rheumatic fever (penicillin) and infective endocarditis (antibiotics before any invasive dental or surgical procedure); treat atrial fibrillation with digitalis or beta-blockers to control ventricular rate and warfarin (Coumadin) to reduce the risk of thromboembolic complications, especially in the presence of atrial fibrillation; for severe disease, consider valvuloplasty versus surgical replacement of the valve; complications include pulmonary hypertension, CHF, atrial fibrillation, infective endocarditis, and systemic thromboembolic phenomena.

ID/CC	A 79-year-old female complains of **severe shortness of breath** (= DYSPNEA) at rest.
HPI	The patient states that she suffered an **MI** one year ago. Since then she **needs three pillows to sleep** (= ORTHOPNEA) and sometimes **wakes up at night coughing** with shortness of breath (= PAROXYSMAL NOCTURNAL DYSPNEA). Additionally, she notes a loss of appetite (= ANOREXIA).
PE	VS: **tachycardia** (HR 130); **tachypnea** (RR 34); **normal BP.** PE: in acute distress; diaphoretic; cyanosis; **JVD; bilateral rales;** PMI displaced downward and to left; S3 and S4 heard; **tender hepatomegaly; pedal edema.**
Labs	LFTs: mildly elevated hepatic enzymes (due to hepatic congestion). ECG: Q waves in V1–V4 (old anterior wall MI); ST elevation in leads V5–V6 (acute lateral wall ischemia).
Imaging	**[A]** CXR: cardiomegaly; prominent pulmonary vasculature; interstitial pulmonary edema. **[B]** CXR: **Kerley B** lines are found in the peripheral lung bases and are manifestations of interstitial pulmonary edema. **[C]** CXR: Kerley A lines are seen more toward the lung apices. Echo: akinetic anterior wall; LV ejection fraction 30%.
Pathogenesis	Congestive heart failure (CHF) represents a syndrome characterized by inability of the heart to provide adequate output to meet the metabolic demands of the body tissues as a result of **systolic or diastolic dysfunction.** Systolic dysfunction arises in conditions that lead to decreased contractility (MI, toxic cardiomyopathy) or increased afterload (severe chronic hypertension, dilated cardiomyopathy, and aortic stenosis). Conversely, diastolic dysfunction arises as a result of impaired active (myocardial ischemia, ventricular hypertrophy) or passive (amyloidosis, constrictive pericarditis) relaxation.
Epidemiology	Annually, > 750,000 individuals die from heart disease. Approximately 90% of these deaths are attributable to **ischemic heart disease, hypertensive heart disease and cor pulmonale,** valvular disease, and congenital disease. CHF is the final common pathway of these conditions.

CONGESTIVE HEART FAILURE

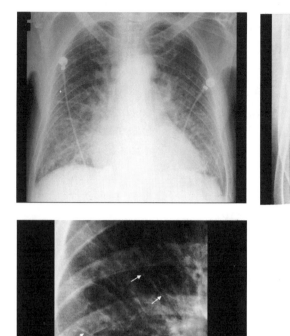

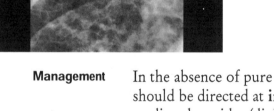

Management	In the absence of pure diastolic dysfunction, therapy should be directed at **increasing contractility** with cardiac glycosides (digitalis), beta-adrenergic agonists, and phosphodiesterase inhibitors. **Reduction of preload and afterload** (ACE inhibitors are considered the first line of therapy for systolic dysfunction) may also improve symptoms. When pulmonary edema is present, oxygen, diuretics, morphine, and vasodilators are frequently indicated; however, these measures provide only symptomatic relief. Ideally, therapy should also be directed toward treating the underlying etiology of the CHF. A low-salt diet is primarily used to control fluid overload.
Complications	Hypoxic encephalopathy, prerenal azotemia, and death.
Associated Diseases	◻ **Chronic Obstructive Pulmonary Disease** Obstruction to airflow, particularly in small airways, due to emphysema, chronic bronchitis, or chronic asthma, commonly in smokers; presents with a predominantly emphysematous (characterized by marked dyspnea, barrel-shaped chest), predominantly bronchitic (characterized by chronic productive cough,

cyanosis, polycythemia, right heart failure), or combined symptomatology; hypoxia, hypercapnia, and polycythemia; CXR shows lung hyperinflation; $FEV_1/FVC < 80\%$ of predicted; treat with smoking cessation, home oxygen, albuterol inhaler, corticosteroids, antibiotics during acute exacerbations; complications include pulmonary hypertension leading to cor pulmonale.

◻ **Nephrotic Syndrome** A clinical complex characterized by proteinuria of > 3.5 g per 1.73 m^2 per 24 hr (in practice, > 3.0–3.5 g per 24 hr), hypoalbuminemia, edema, hyperlipidemia, lipiduria, and hypercoagulability; six entities account for $> 90\%$ of cases: minimal change disease (most common cause in children), focal and segmental glomerulosclerosis, membranous glomerulopathy (most common cause in adults), membranoproliferative glomerulonephritis, diabetic nephropathy, and amyloidosis; presents with lower extremity swelling, periorbital edema, and ascites; renal biopsies show different patterns on light, immunofluorescence, and electron microscopy; treatments vary depending on subtype; in general, corticosteroids, cyclophosphamide, azathioprine, or cyclosporine may be used; ascites is treated with fluid and salt restriction and diuretics; renal transplantation should be considered for severe disease or end-stage renal disease.

ID/CC	A 60-year-old male presents with progressive, **severe shortness of breath** (= DYSPNEA) and **cough.**
HPI	The patient is a **chronic smoker** and has been receiving treatment for **COPD.** He reports **swollen feet** and an increase in **abdominal girth.**
PE	VS: tachycardia (HR 120); tachypnea (RR 30); weight gain (due to fluid retention); hypoxia (SaO_2 88% on room air). PE: moderate **respiratory distress;** central cyanosis present; **JVP elevated;** bilateral pitting **pedal edema; bilateral rhonchi and crepitations,** the character of which changes with coughing; palpable left parasternal heave; loud P2 and **RV S3;** ascites and mildly **tender hepatomegaly.**
Labs	ABGs: **hypoxia and respiratory alkalosis.** CBC: elevated hematocrit (55). ECG: right axis deviation; **P pulmonale;** RVH.
Imaging	**[A]** CXR: enlargement of the hilar vasculature; prominence of the main pulmonary artery; relative cardiomegaly given the degree of hyperinflation. **[B]** CXR: another case, again showing a massive main pulmonary artery and cardiomegaly. Echo: **RV dilatation.** US-Abdomen: **congestive hepatomegaly** and ascites.
Pathogenesis	Cor pulmonale is defined as enlargement of the right ventricle secondary to diseases of the lungs, thorax, or pulmonary circulation. Pulmonary hypertension eventually increases RV afterload, and ultimately results in RV failure. Although the most common cause is COPD, other causes include primary pulmonary hypertension, chronic bronchitis, recurrent pulmonary embolism, sickle cell anemia, interstitial lung disease, bronchiectasis, chronic bronchial asthma, cystic fibrosis, myasthenia gravis, ankylosing spondylitis, and vasculitis.
Epidemiology	Cor pulmonale is a common condition owing to its association with COPD.
Management	**Correct alveolar hypoxia** by judiciously **increasing the inspired O_2 concentration** (ventilation is in part driven by hypoxia in these patients) and improving alveolar ventilation by relieving the airway obstruction **(bronchodilators and steroids). Diuretics** relieve the

COR PULMONALE

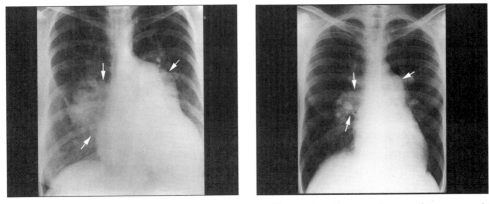

edema. **Restrict sodium intake; quit smoking;** avoid alcohol and sedatives.

Complications

Supraventricular or ventricular arrhythmias and biventricular cardiac failure are common complications.

Associated Diseases

◘ **Chronic Bronchitis** A form of COPD marked by bronchial wall thickening and excessive mucus production due to smoking, chronic asthma, or chronic inhalation of other irritants; presents with productive cough for > 3 months in a year for > 2 consecutive years, progressive exertional dyspnea, and cyanosis; severe hypoxia, polycythemia, and hypercapnia; FEV_1/FVC < 80% of predicted; CXR may reveal pulmonary hypertension and cardiomegaly; treat with oxygen supplementation, bronchodilators, antibiotics, smoking cessation, and corticosteroids; complications include pulmonary hypertension leading to cor pulmonale.

◘ **Emphysema** A form of COPD marked by alveolar destruction; caused by smoking (centroacinar emphysema) or, more rarely, alpha-antitrypsin deficiency (panacinar emphysema); presents with cough, dyspnea, characteristic puffing of the lips during expiration to elevate airway pressures, and barrel-shaped chest; hypercapnia and hypoxia; FEV_1/FVC < 80% of predicted; CXR reveals elongated tubular heart shadow and lung hyperinflation with flat diaphragms; treat with home oxygen and smoking cessation; complications include pulmonary hypertension leading to cor pulmonale.

◘ **Primary Pulmonary Hypertension** An idiopathic

increase in pulmonary artery pressure and pulmonary vascular resistance; seen in young women; presents with progressive dyspnea refractory to oxygen therapy, large "a" wave in JVP, and loud P2; polycythemia; ECG shows right axis deviation and right ventricular and atrial hypertrophy; treat with prostacyclin, calcium channel blockers, adenosine or nitric oxide; consider heart-lung transplantation before disease progresses to cor pulmonale.

ID/CC	A 50-year-old male experiences progressive **shortness of breath** and pronounced intolerance of physical activity.
HPI	He also complains of cough and swelling of his ankles. He is in his seventh month of chemotherapy (including **daunorubicin**) for non-Hodgkin's lymphoma.
PE	VS: tachycardia; mild hypotension (BP 100/60); tachypnea. PE: respiratory distress; faint rales heard bilaterally; **elevated JVP; holosystolic murmur** in mitral and tricuspid areas; **2+ pitting edema** in lower extremities.
Labs	CBC: normal. **Increased BUN and creatinine;** BUN/creatinine ratio > 20 (sign of prerenal azotemia). Lytes: **hyponatremia.**
Imaging	CXR: sinus tachycardia with cardiomegaly. **[A]** Echo: LV (1) and RV (2) dilatation and systolic dysfunction (reduced EF).
Pathogenesis	Most cases of dilated cardiomyopathy are **idiopathic;** other causes include **long-standing hypertension, alcohol abuse, beriberi, coxsackievirus** infection, and **cocaine abuse.** In this case, heart failure was most likely secondary to chemotherapy with **daunorubicin.** Dilated cardiomyopathy usually presents clinically as CHF secondary to diminished LV function and decreased CO.
Epidemiology	Most cases are sporadic. Twenty percent of patients demonstrate familial forms with various modes of genetic transmission.
Management	Bed rest and **supportive care.** Use diuretics, ACE inhibitors, vasodilators (nitrates), and digitalis to treat CHF; control total body sodium and volume. Consider oral anticoagulation due to the high risk of atrial and ventricular arrhythmia. Immunosuppressive therapy may be tried; primary valvular disease and CAD should be managed. Consider **cardiac transplantation. Immunize** against influenza and pneumococcal pneumonia. Identify and treat reversible causes of dilated cardiomyopathy (alcohol abuse, pregnancy, selenium deficiency, hypophosphatemia, hypocalcemia, thyroid disease, cocaine use, and chronic uncontrolled tachycardia).
Complications	Complications include deterioration of ventricular

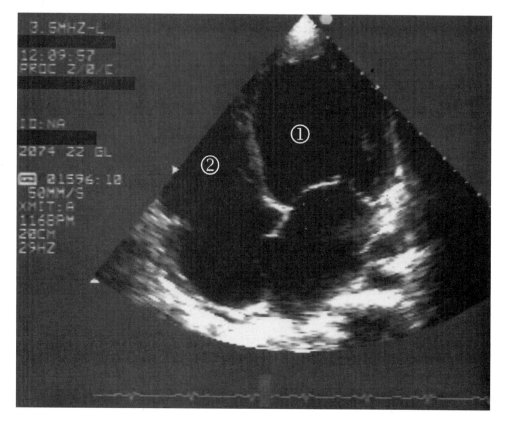

function followed by death (due to **arrhythmias** or **intractable CHF**). Systemic and pulmonary thromboembolic complications may also occur.

Associated Diseases

■ **Congestive Heart Failure** Failure of cardiac output to meet the metabolic demands of the body due to a deficit in myocardial contractility or an increase in workload; a common complication of ischemic and hypertensive heart disease in the elderly; presents with orthopnea, paroxysmal nocturnal dyspnea, exertional dyspnea, weight loss, pedal edema, neck vein distention, third heart sound, and pulmonary rales; echo reveals decreased cardiac output and ejection fraction; treat with bed rest, propped-up position, oxygen, fluid and salt restriction, preload reduction (with venodilators and diuretics), after-load reduction (with arteriolar dilators), and measures to increase cardiac contractility (with digitalis, beta-adrenergic agonists, and amrinone).

■ **Hypertrophic Cardiomyopathy** Ventricular outflow tract obstruction by hypertrophy; an autosomal-dominant inheritance pattern is seen in almost half of all cases; presents with dyspnea on exertion, angina,

DILATED CARDIOMYOPATHY

syncope, and even sudden death (commonly associated with strenuous physical activity) on presentation; ECG shows LVH; echo shows asymmetrical septal hypertrophy, systolic anterior motion of the mitral valve, and mitral regurgitation; treat with avoidance of competitive sports and strenuous physical activity, negative inotropic agents (beta-blockers and calcium channel blockers), amiodarone, possible surgical myomectomy of the interventricular septum.

◘ **Restrictive Cardiomyopathy** Fibrosis of myocardium characterized by impaired diastolic filling with preserved contractile function, usually secondary to scleroderma, amyloidosis, sarcoidosis, hemachromatosis, or storage disorders (e.g., Fabry's disease); presents with dyspnea, orthopnea, peripheral edema, distended neck veins, and audible S4; ECG shows low voltage; CXR reveals normal-sized cardiac shadow; myocardial biopsy demonstrates disease within myocardium; treat the underlying condition; cardiac transplantation is the only effective treatment for cardiac disease once it has begun; without transplant, five-year survival is poor.

ID/CC	A **20-year-old** male is brought to the ER after collapsing during a tennis match.
HPI	He states that his father was forced to quit his college basketball team after episodes of syncope.
PE	VS: **hypertension** (BP 168/90); **tachycardia** (HR 132); tachypnea. PE: brisk carotid upstroke with palpable double impulse; **double apical cardiac impulse,** prominent S4, and **coarse systolic outflow murmur** localized along left sternal border and accentuated by the Valsalva maneuver.
Labs	ECG: left axis deviation (due to LVH) and right bundle branch block. Muscle biopsy reveals myocardial disarray.
Imaging	CXR: evidence of left atrial and ventricular enlargement. Echo: increased thickness of the ventricular septum.
Pathogenesis	Hypertrophic obstructive cardiomyopathy is characterized by the presence of **heterogenous LVH** (usually with preferential LV septal hypertrophy) in association with a **dynamic LV outflow tract pressure gradient** (due to midsystolic apposition of the anterior mitral valve leaflet against the hypertrophic septum, resulting in a subaortic narrowing). Decreased compliance of the hypertrophic muscle results in elevated diastolic filling pressures, leading to diastolic dysfunction.
Epidemiology	A genetic component (with **autosomal-dominant** inheritance) has been observed in about half of all cases. A common cause of sudden death in young athletes.
Management	Key management components include avoidance of strenuous physical activity; beta-blockers (to reduce heart rate and blood pressure); calcium channel blockers, particularly verapamil and diltiazem (to augment diastolic ventricular filling); and surgery (septal myomectomy) for cases that are unresponsive to medical therapy.
Complications	Atrial fibrillation, systemic embolization, sudden death, and infective endocarditis.
Associated Diseases	◻ **Aortic Stenosis** Stenosis of the aortic valve commonly due to congenital bicuspid valves, progressive

7. **HYPERTROPHIC OBSTRUCTIVE CARDIOMYOPATHY**

senile calcification of normal valve, or rheumatic heart disease; presents with angina, exertional dyspnea, and syncope; crescendo-decrescendo systolic ejection murmur over the right second intercostal space radiating to the carotids; paradoxical splitting of S2; treat with balloon valvuloplasty, surgical valve replacement; complications include CHF.

HYPERTROPHIC OBSTRUCTIVE CARDIOMYOPATHY

ID/CC	A 65-year-old man with end-stage prostate cancer develops **dyspnea on exertion.**
HPI	He has a 25-pack-year smoking history. He was diagnosed with **prostate cancer** at age 62. Aggressive therapy was abandoned two months ago.
PE	VS: **wide pulse pressure** (BP 146/52); **tachycardia** (HR 112); bounding pulses; tachypnea. PE: **diastolic murmur** localized at right sternal border; full hard pulse followed by sudden collapse (= CORRIGAN'S PULSE); rhythmical nodding of head synchronous with heartbeat (= DE MUSSET'S SIGN); loud "pistol shot" heard on auscultation over femoral arteries (= TRAUBE'S SIGN) (signs of aortic insufficiency).
Labs	CBC/Lytes: normal. Blood cultures negative.
Imaging	N/A
Pathogenesis	Marantic endocarditis is characteristically associated with terminal illnesses such as metastatic cancer (commonly adenocarcinomas and promyelocytic leukemia). Pathologically, cardiac valves reveal the presence of small, **sterile fibrin deposits** (vegetations) distributed along their lines of closure.
Epidemiology	N/A
Management	Aortic valve replacement is not indicated because the patient has end-stage cancer. Therapy should be directed toward minimization of symptoms. Prevention involves treatment of underlying cause—in this case, prostate cancer.
Complications	Sequelae of valvular heart disease, including CHF.
Associated Diseases	◻ **Bacterial Endocarditis** Infection of prosthetic (usually with *S. epidermidis*), previously diseased (subacute IE, usually with *S. viridans*), or normal (acute IE, as in intravenous drug abusers, usually with *S. aureus*) heart valves; presents with fever, night sweats, and diffuse septic emboli (e.g., brain, kidney, liver, spleen); leukocytosis, elevated ESR, and positive blood cultures; echo reveals valvular vegetations; treat with 4–6 weeks of a penicillin or cephalosporin with or without aminoglycoside; complications include diffuse abscesses, valve destruction with resultant heart failure, and sepsis.

MARANTIC ENDOCARDITIS

◻ **Libman–Sacks Endocarditis** Wartlike valvular vegetations seen in up to 40% of cases of SLE; most often located at the angles of the AV valves or on the ventricular surface of the mitral valve; presents with regurgitant murmurs when associated with anti-phospholipid syndrome, although often asymptomatic; echo may reveal the vegetations; treat underlying SLE, anticoagulate.

◻ **Prosthetic Valve Endocarditis** Infection of the heart valves after surgery; when presenting within two months of surgery it is commonly caused by *Staphylococcus epidermidis* or fungal contamination of wound site; later presentations are caused by viridans group streptococci, *Staphylococcus epidermidis*, or fastidious gram-negative rods; presents with subacute onset of fever, night sweats with diffuse embolic disease, and heart murmur; elevated ESR; echo reveals valvular vegetation; treat with surgical replacement of valve and 4–6 weeks of a penicillin or cephalosporin, rifampin with or without aminoglycoside; complications include valve dehiscence.

ID/CC	A 56-year-old male who suffered an acute non-Q-wave anterolateral MI is found to have a new murmur during his third day in the CCU.
HPI	He has a history of CAD. He was admitted for severe precordial chest pain that lasted for five hours. On day three he began to complain of increasing dyspnea and fatigue.
PE	VS: hypertension (BP 148/83). PE: in mild distress; brisk carotid upstroke; diffuse bibasilar rales; prominent S3 and S4; **III/VI pansystolic murmur best heard at the apex with radiation to the axilla;** hyperdynamic LV impulse; distal pulses intact; no peripheral edema.
Labs	CBC/Lytes: normal. CPK elevated; CK-MB fraction elevated; mildly elevated troponin I; Swan–Ganz catheter was placed, demonstrating **no step-up in blood oxygen saturation** from right atrium to pulmonary artery; giant V waves (corresponding to ventricular systole) noted on pressure tracings. ECG: left atrial enlargement.
Imaging	Echo: flail mitral leaflet with papillary muscle rupture. **[A]** CXR: another case showing massive enlargement of the right heart border (1), prominence of the main pulmonary artery, and calcification of the mitral valve (2). **[B]** CXR: another case showing "cephalization" (upper zone vessels are larger than equivalent vessels in the lower lung zones).
Pathogenesis	Mitral valve insufficiency is most commonly secondary to myxomatous degeneration (mitral valve prolapse), valve perforation (infective endocarditis), subvalvular dysfunction (papillary muscle dysfunction or ruptured chordae tendineae due to acute MI), rheumatic heart disease (once the most common cause), or, rarely, cardiac tumors (left atrial myxoma).
Epidemiology	N/A
Management	Proper management relies on **accurate identification of the underlying cause.** Doppler studies provide both qualitative and semi-quantitative estimates of mitral regurgitation severity. Cardiac catheterization provides accurate assessment of regurgitation, LV function, and pulmonary artery pressures. Coronary angiography defines underlying coronary disease present prior to

MITRAL INSUFFICIENCY

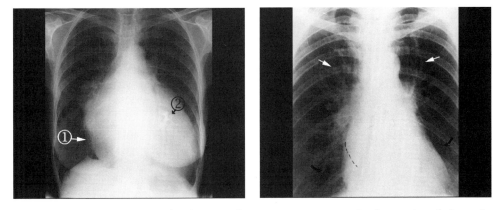

valvular repair. **Emergent surgical repair** of the mitral valve is often indicated in cases of acute mitral regurgitation due to MI, endocarditis, or ruptured chordae tendineae. Chronic mitral insufficiency may remain asymptomatic for years and may require surgical repair only upon progressive deterioration of LV function or when disease becomes activity-limiting.

Complications

Mitral insufficiency is a risk factor for atrial fibrillation and infective endocarditis. Patients with mitral valve prolapse should receive antibiotic prophylaxis prior to dental and surgical procedures. Supraventricular tachycardias can be controlled with beta-blockers. Ventricular tachycardias (and sudden death) are rare and require anti-arrhythmic therapy. Mitral valve prolapse is associated with increased embolic cerebrovascular events.

Associated Diseases

◘ **Marfan's Syndrome** An autosomal-dominant defect in the fibrillin protein, which is required for collagen-fibril stability; presents with classic marfanoid features (tall, thin patients with long digits), cardiac valvular disease (mitral valve prolapse, mitral and aortic regurgitation), lenticular dislocation, and joint laxity; treatment is supportive; complications include cardiac disease.

◘ **Embolic Stroke** Emboli most commonly from the carotid or heart; presents with focal neurologic deficit, often presaged by reversible neurologic deficits (= TIA); head CT or MR demonstrates infarction; carotid US may show atherosclerotic stenosis; treat with tPA if the patient presents soon after symptom onset (contraindicated if hemorrhagic stroke); continue long-term anticoagulation; perform endarterectomy if carotid stenosis > 70%; attempt conversion of atrial fibrillation to normal sinus rhythm; complications include cerebral edema, herniation, and hemorrhage.

MITRAL INSUFFICIENCY

ID/CC	A 35-year-old **female** presents with **hemoptysis** and **dyspnea on exertion.**
HPI	She reports a childhood history of fever accompanied by joint pain and skin rash **(acute rheumatic fever)**; since that time she has been diagnosed with a valvular heart disease and has been receiving penicillin injections every three weeks.
PE	VS: low-volume pulse. PE: mild peripheral cyanosis (due to reduced cardiac output); left parasternal heave; loud S1 and P2; **"rumbling" mid-diastolic murmur** with presystolic accentuation heard at apex; opening snap (OS) heard at apex; A2–OS interval short (severe mitral stenosis).
Labs	ECG: P mitrale; RVH.
Imaging	**[A]** CXR: left atrial enlargement (1); pulmonary venous congestion. **[B]** Barium Swallow: narrowing of the esophagus by enlarged left atrium. Echo: fusion of commissures causes the posterior leaflet to move anteriorly with the anterior leaflet rather than in its usual posterior direction during diastole. M-Mode Echo: flattening of E-F slope. The mitral valve orifice is calculated to be $< 1 \text{ cm}^2$ (critical mitral stenosis).
Pathogenesis	Mitral stenosis is generally rheumatic in origin; rarely it may be congenital (e.g., ASD with acquired mitral stenosis–Lutembacher syndrome). Mitral stenosis and mitral insufficiency often coexist.
Epidemiology	Two-thirds of all patients with mitral stenosis are females. Pure or predominant mitral stenosis occurs in approximately 40% of all patients with rheumatic heart disease. The occurrence of mitral stenosis is decreasing in developed countries owing to the declining incidence of rheumatic fever.
Management	**Because mitral stenosis is usually asymptomatic for many years, no treatment may be required for a long time.** Pregnancy (increased cardiac output and transmural pressure gradient) or atrial fibrillation may precipitate severe symptoms. Patients with **atrial fibrillation** should be converted to and maintained in sinus rhythm with **digoxin or antiarrhythmics** and should be given **warfarin** anticoagulation to prevent

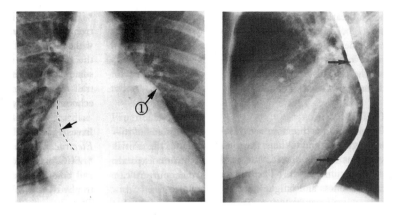

embolic events. Most patients do not require **surgical therapy** until they develop (1) recalcitrant pulmonary edema; (2) activity-limiting dyspnea and pulmonary edema; (3) pulmonary hypertension with RVH or hemoptysis; (4) activity limitation despite ventricular rate control and medical therapy; or (5) recurrent systemic emboli despite anticoagulation. **Open mitral valve commissurotomy** is effective in most patients in the absence of substantial regurgitation. **Balloon valvuloplasty** is an increasingly common procedure for patients without regurgitation. **Valve replacement** is the definitive treatment; it is performed for critical mitral stenosis, mitral incompetence, calcified valves, left atrial thrombus, and floppy valves. All patients with rheumatic heart disease should receive **prophylactic antibiotics** prior to dental, surgical, and urologic procedures to prevent endocarditis. Women with known disease should be counseled regarding the risks associated with pregnancy.

Complications

Patients may develop pulmonary hypertension, right heart failure, atrial fibrillation, systemic and cerebral embolization, and bacterial endocarditis.

Associated Diseases

◘ **Left Atrial Myxoma** The most common primary cardiac tumor; occurs in middle age; presents with dizziness, syncope, fever, recurrent systemic emboli, weight loss, and a low-pitched early to mid-diastolic sound that is variable with position (= TUMOR PLOP); echo shows mass in atrium; treat with surgical excision.

◘ **Rheumatic Fever** Complication of group A streptococcal infection, secondary to autoantibodies directed against joints and heart valves; presents > 1 week after throat infection with migratory polyarthritis, endocarditis, and rash; antistreptococcal antibodies (e.g., ASO); treat with aspirin and penicillin; complications include permanent valvular disease.

ID/CC	A **58-year-old male** complains of **oppressive retrosternal pain** that **radiates to the jaw and left arm;** the pain has lasted **more than 30 minutes.**
HPI	He also complains of **shortness of breath, nausea,** and extreme **fatigue.** He has **hypertension,** is **obese,** and has **elevated serum cholesterol** levels.
PE	VS: **hypotension** (BP 82/48); **tachycardia** (HR 110); tachypnea. PE: obese; **acute distress;** profusely **diaphoretic;** increased JVP; **basilar rales; S4** heard best in left lateral recumbency.
Labs	CBC: leukocytosis. **Increased troponin T and I** (initial elevation within first 8 hours) and **CK-MB** (initial elevation within first 24 hours). ECG: ST elevation; Q waves; inverted T waves in leads V1 to V4 consistent with an **anterior** infarct (lateral infarct in I and aVL; inferior infarct in II, III, and aVF; posterior infarct will show ST depression and larger R waves in V1 and V2).
Imaging	CXR: normal. Echo: decreased wall motion.
Pathogenesis	A localized area of myocardial **necrosis** caused by reduced blood flow below the level necessary for cell viability, usually caused by **atherosclerosis** of coronary arteries. Other causes include coronary artery aneurysms, arteritis, spasm, cocaine overdose, and cyanide or carbon monoxide poisoning.
Epidemiology	Ischemic heart disease is the leading cause of death in the U.S., followed by cancer; it usually occurs in males > 50 years and in postmenopausal women. It may present as myocardial infarction, sudden death, CHF, or chronic angina. In the U.S. there are > 500,000 myocardial infarctions each year.
Management	Initial management includes **oxygen, aspirin, nitroglycerin** (sublingual or transdermal), **morphine,** and a **beta-blocker** unless contraindicated. Definitive therapy is aimed at restoring perfusion to the ischemic area as soon as possible. This is accomplished by emergent cardiac catheterization with **balloon angioplasty** (if immediately available) or intravenous **thrombolytic** infusion (unless contraindicated). Start IV **heparin** and admit the patient to the CCU for **continuous ECG monitoring.** Give ACE inhibitors

MYOCARDIAL INFARCTION

for those with an EF < 40%.

Complications   **Arrhythmias** (most common cause of death in early post-MI period; usually ventricular fibrillation), pulmonary edema, heart failure, ventricular aneurysm formation, cardiogenic shock, mitral insufficiency, mural thrombosis and embolism, pericarditis (3–5 days post-MI), ventricular wall or papillary muscle rupture (5–10 days post-MI), and post-MI pericarditis (= DRESSLER'S SYNDROME) (probably an autoimmune process occurring 1–12 weeks post-MI). **FIRST AID 2** p. 64

Associated Diseases   ◻ **Acute Pericarditis** Inflammation of the pericardium, most commonly caused by viral infection (coxsackievirus, echovirus, adenovirus); other causes include bacterial, tubercular, and fungal infections, uremia, malignant infiltration (breast/lung carcinoma, Hodgkin's lymphoma), and post-irradiation or postmyocardial injury; presents with characteristic chest pain that decreases on sitting up and leaning forward; triphasic pericardial rub heard on auscultation; ECG reveals diffuse ST-segment elevation and T-wave inversion; echo may reveal small pericardial effusion; treat with NSAIDs; complications include cardiac tamponade and constrictive pericarditis.

◻ **Prinzmetal's Angina** Idiopathic coronary artery spasm; usually affects women < 50 years; presents with recurrent attacks of severe retrosternal crushing pain occurring at rest; during the attack, ECG shows ST-segment elevations; treat with sublingual nitroglycerin for acute pain relief, calcium channel blockers for long-term prophylaxis; complications include arrhythmia or sudden death.

◻ **Unstable Angina** Cardiac ischemic chest pain occurring at rest or showing an increase from typical angina patterns; ECG shows ST-segment depression and T-wave flattening; treat with urgent heparinization and coronary angioplasty; complications include a high risk of subsequent myocardial infarction.

ID/CC	A 25-year-old female presents complaining of **syncope**, excessive anxiety, and **palpitations.**
HPI	She is taking verapamil daily for a heart condition.
PE	VS: tachycardia (HR 150); hypotension (BP 90/50). PE: JVP normal; normal S1 and S2; remainder of systemic exam normal.
Labs	ECG: **narrow QRS complexes without preceding P waves** (suggestive of AV nodal reentrant tachycardia).
Imaging	CXR: normal.
Pathogenesis	Most cases of paroxysmal supraventricular tachycardia are caused by **reentry** at one of three sites: (1) in the AV node in about 40%–50% of cases; (2) over a concealed, extranodal accessory bypass tract in 30%–40% of cases; and (3) in the sinus node or atria in 5%–10% of cases.
Epidemiology	The condition is very common and is often experienced by people with structurally normal hearts. It is frequently seen in preexcitation syndromes and in association with certain congenital abnormalities, such as ASD and Ebstein's anomaly. It also occurs in patients with rheumatic, atherosclerotic, hypertensive, or thyrotoxic heart disease; may occur following MI; and may be precipitated by stress, tobacco, caffeine, or alcohol.
Management	Treatment is aimed at blocking AV node conduction, including the use of **vagal maneuvers** for acute attacks (e.g., carotid sinus massage). If unsuccessful, attempt pharmacologic therapy. **IV adenosine** is currently the drug of choice because of its short half-life. **IV verapamil** is also considered a first-line agent. Beta-blockers are second-line agents and should not be used concurrently with calcium channel blockers (may cause sinus arrest or severe hypotension). **Digoxin** should not be used acutely because of its prolonged onset of action. **Cardioversion is the initial treatment of choice when there is marked hypotension,** severe angina, or cardiovascular collapse or when pharmacologic measures fail; do not use when digitalis toxicity is suspected. **Radiofrequency catheter ablation** is now the treatment of choice for long-term suppression in patients with symptomatic

PAROXYSMAL SUPRAVENTRICULAR TACHYCARDIA

supraventricular tachycardias associated with manifest accessory atrioventricular pathways (e.g., Wolff–Parkinson–White syndrome), concealed accessory atrioventricular pathways, and AV nodal reentry. Pharmacologic therapies for the chronic suppression of paroxysmal supraventricular tachycardia include calcium channel blockers, beta-blockers, and digoxin.

Complications

LV failure may result from coexistent structural heart disease. Complications also include ventricular arrhythmias.

Associated Diseases

◘ **Atrial Flutter** Arrhythmia due to an ectopic impulse in the atrium; presents with palpitations, although often asymptomatic; ECG shows a rate of 250–350 BPM; "sawtooth" pattern best seen in lead II; treat with electrical cardioversion (if hemodynamically unstable), class III antiarrhythmic agents.

◘ **Atrial Fibrillation** The most common chronic arrhythmia; causes include mitral valve disease, hypertensive and ischemic heart disease, dilated cardiomyopathy, alcoholism, and hyperthyroidism; presents with irregularly irregular pulse, palpitations, and dyspnea; ECG shows no discernible P waves; treat with beta-blockers, calcium channel blockers, or digitalis to control ventricular rate, warfarin (Coumadin) to prevent mural thrombi; can attempt cardioversion with class IA or IC antiarrhythmic agents or DC shock.

◘ **Multifocal Atrial Tachycardia** Tachycardia caused by multiple coexisting cardiac pacemakers; commonly seen in chronic lung disease or theophylline toxicity; presents with palpitations or can be asymptomatic; ECG shows irregularly irregular pulse with at least three different P-wave morphologies; treat with calcium blockers or digitalis to control ventricular rate; beta-blockers may be contraindicated in lung disease; complications include hemodynamic compromise due to rapid ventricular response.

◘ **Wolff–Parkinson–White Syndrome** Preexcitation syndrome due to the presence of an accessory AV tract (bundle of Kent); associated with certain congenital cardiac defects (Ebstein's anomaly); presents with episodic syncope, angina, and palpitations; ECG shows short PR interval and wide QRS complex with a slurred upstroke (= DELTA WAVE); may also reveal reentrant tachycardias as paroxysmal supraventricular tachycardia (PSVT), atrial flutter, or atrial fibrillation; treat definitively with catheter radiofrequency ablation of bypass tract, medical management of narrow complex reentry tachycardias (PSVT, atrial flutter, atrial fibrillation) with adenosine, verapamil, or DC cardioversion (if hemodynamically unstable).

12.   PAROXYSMAL SUPRAVENTRICULAR TACHYCARDIA

ID/CC	A 27-year-old female presents with **chest pain** and low-grade **fever** of one week's duration.
HPI	Her **retrosternal pain** is relieved somewhat when she sits up and leans forward.
PE	VS: normal. PE: normal pulse with regular rhythm; triphasic, high-pitched scratching sound heard over left lower sternal border (= PERICARDIAL FRICTION RUB).
Labs	**[A]** ECG: **PR segment depression and diffuse ST-segment elevation;** later stages show inverted T waves without Q waves.
Imaging	**[B]** Echo: good cardiac function with small pericardial effusion. CXR: normal.
Pathogenesis	Viral infections (**coxsackie B,** echo, HIV) are the most common cause of acute pericarditis. Other causes include bacterial infections (pneumococcus, staphylococcus, meningococcus, *Mycobacterium tuberculosis,* and *H. influenzae*); fungal infections (*Histoplasma capsulatum*); uremia; drug-induced pericarditis (procainamide and minoxidil); radiation-induced pericardial effusion (common in patients who have received large doses of radiation to the mediastinum); neoplasms (most often with breast or lung cancer); post-cardiac surgery or postcardiotomy syndrome; and post-MI immune-mediated pericarditis (= DRESSLER'S SYNDROME).
Epidemiology	The incidence of tuberculous pericarditis and other forms of bacterial pericarditis in the U.S. is increasing as a result of the AIDS epidemic.
Management	Manage acute idiopathic or viral pericarditis with **NSAIDs.** Malignant pericardial effusion can often be managed palliatively with pericardiocentesis, placement of pericardial window, radiotherapy, or chemotherapy. Purulent pericarditis requires **pericardiocentesis and IV antibiotics.** Monitor for cardiac tamponade or constrictive pericarditis. Avoid anticoagulants in light of the risk of precipitating hemorrhagic effusion.
Complications	Complications include **cardiac tamponade. Constrictive pericarditis** results from fibrosis of the pericardial sac, most commonly due to progression of active tuberculous pericarditis.

PERICARDITIS

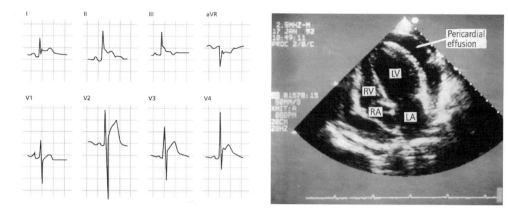

I	II	III	aVR
V1	V2	V3	V4

Pericardial effusion

LV
RV
RA
LA

Associated Diseases

☐ **Constrictive Pericarditis** Fibrosis of the pericardium during resolution of acute pericarditis caused by tuberculosis, viral infection, collagen vascular disease, malignancy (breast or lymphoma), or post-trauma or myocardial infarction; presents with distended neck veins, hepatosplenomegaly with ascites, pulsus paradoxus, orthopnea, and exertional dyspnea; central venous and pulmonary artery pressures are elevated; ECG shows low voltage; echo and CT may reveal calcified, thickened pericardium; treat with pericardiectomy.

☐ **Pericardial Effusion** Fluid within the pericardial sac; may be idiopathic or associated with pericarditis of any etiology; presents with fatigue, dyspnea, chest pain, and faint heart sounds; ECG reveals low-voltage electrical alternans; echo demonstrates the presence of effusion; treat with pericardiocentesis if the effusion is large enough to compromise cardiac output; treat the underlying disorder; complications include cardiac tamponade leading to hemodynamic compromise.

☐ **Systemic Lupus Erythematosus** A systemic autoimmune disease primarily affecting young women; more common in blacks; presents with malar skin rash, nephritis, neurologic disease, photosensitivity, protean organ dysfunction, serositis, and arthritis; ANA positive; anti-dsDNA more specific but less sensitive; antiphospholipid antibodies in certain types; treat with NSAIDs, corticosteroids, cyclophosphamide if necessary.

ID/CC	A 26-year-old female presents with increasing **shortness of breath** over the past month.
HPI	As a teenager, she had a prior episode of **rheumatic fever** with no known cardiac or pulmonary disease. She has recently had symptoms of **orthopnea** and several episodes of **paroxysmal nocturnal dyspnea**.
PE	VS: normal. PE: no acute distress; lungs clear; S1 (prominent) and S2; mild precordial bulge; **short II/VI diastolic murmur and IV/VI low-pitched rumbling presystolic murmur at lower left sternal border and apex with loud mid-diastolic opening snap; presystolic thrill appreciated at apex.**
Labs	ECG: tall, peaked P waves in limb leads and broad negative phases of diphasic P in V1; right axis deviation indicating RVH.
Imaging	CXR: enlarged left atrium; elevated left main stem bronchus; large pulmonary artery in the presence of pulmonary hypertension. Echo: thickened, immobile mitral valve with anterior and posterior leaflets moving together (rather than in opposite directions); slow early diastolic filling slope; left atrial enlargement; decreased valve area (< 1.5 cm^2). US **(doppler)**: prolonged pressure half-time across the mitral valve and indirect markers of pulmonary hypertension.
Pathogenesis	Rheumatic heart disease occurs as a late sequela of rheumatic fever, usually arising many years following the initial episode. The pathologic process represents an immunologic response to **streptococcal** antigens in which a **multisystem inflammatory cascade** is triggered with characteristic inflammation of the pericardium, myocardium, and endocardium. Endocarditis, valvular thickening, fibrosis, and prominent calcification occur in areas subject to greatest hemodynamic stress. The **mitral valve is most frequently involved** (50%–60% of cases), but the aortic valve is also commonly affected (often in combination with mitral disease); tricuspid involvement is rare ($< 10\%$ and almost always in association with mitral and aortic disease), and the pulmonary valve is almost never affected.
Epidemiology	In developed countries, the near-elimination of rheumatic fever has resulted in a dramatic decrease in

new cases of rheumatic heart disease. However, rheumatic heart disease continues to be the most common underlying cause of mitral stenosis in the elderly. A history of rheumatic fever is found in only 60% of patients with rheumatic heart disease. Following the initial episode of rheumatic fever, immediate mortality is 1%–2%; nevertheless, 80% of affected children reach adulthood, and only half have any limitation of activity secondary to valvular disease. Rheumatic heart disease remains prevalent in the developing world.

Management

Management is dependent on the specific valvular involvement. **Mitral stenosis** is **usually asymptomatic with minimal limitation in activity for many years.** Pregnancy (increased cardiac output and transmural pressure gradient) or atrial fibrillation may precipitate severe symptoms. Patients with atrial fibrillation should be converted to and maintained in sinus rhythm with digoxin or antiarrhythmics and should be given warfarin anticoagulation to prevent embolic events. Most patients do not require surgical therapy until they develop (1) recalcitrant pulmonary edema; (2) activity-limiting dyspnea and pulmonary edema; (3) pulmonary hypertension with RVH or hemoptysis; (4) activity limitation despite ventricular rate control and medical therapy; or (5) recurrent systemic emboli despite anticoagulation. **Open mitral valve commissurotomy** is effective in most patients in the absence of substantial regurgitation. **Balloon valvuloplasty** is an increasingly common procedure for patients without regurgitation. **Valve replacement** is indicated in the presence of significant stenosis, insufficiency, excessive calcification, or destruction that is not amenable to valvulotomy. All patients with rheumatic heart disease should receive **prophylactic antibiotics** prior to dental, surgical, and urologic procedures to prevent endocarditis. Women with known disease should be counseled regarding the risks associated with pregnancy.

Complications

Operative mortality associated with repair procedures is low (1%–3%). Restenosis following surgical repair may occur but is less common with mitral valve repair. Prosthetic valve use is associated with the risk of

RHEUMATIC HEART DISEASE

thrombosis, paravalvular leak, endocarditis, and degenerative valvular changes.

Associated Diseases   ◘ **Mitral Stenosis** Fibrosis of the mitral valve commonly secondary to rheumatic heart disease; presents with dyspnea, hemoptysis, pulmonary edema, mid-diastolic rumble with opening snap at the apex, and RV heave; ECG shows P mitrale (due to left atrial enlargement), RVH, and right axis deviation; echo reveals calcification and stenosed valve orifice; treat with prophylaxis for rheumatic fever (penicillin) and infective endocarditis (antibiotics before any invasive dental or surgical procedure); treat atrial fibrillation with digitalis or beta-blockers to control ventricular rate and warfarin (Coumadin) to reduce the risk of thromboembolic complications, especially in the presence of atrial fibrillation; for severe disease, consider valvuloplasty if the valve is not too heavily calcified; otherwise surgical replacement of the valve; complications include pulmonary hypertension, CHF, atrial fibrillation, infective endocarditis, and systemic thromboembolic phenomena.

ID/CC	A 22-year-old woman presents to the outpatient clinic for follow-up evaluation of elevated blood pressure.
HPI	The patient is an otherwise-healthy, active woman who is involved in long-distance running and biking and has long been on a low-salt, low-fat, low-cholesterol diet. She denies any symptoms or problems. Her previous blood pressure measurements, taken six months and one year ago, were both greater than 150/90. The patient notes that her mother also had high blood pressure, which required medication beginning at an early age.
PE	VS: **hypertension** (BP 150/94). PE: well nourished, muscular, and in no acute distress; HEENT, lung, and cardiac exams normal; abdominal exam remarkable only for soft, audible **epigastric and renal artery bruits.**
Labs	CBC/Lytes: normal. Positive **captopril test** (95% sensitivity and specificity) (administration of captopril results in increase in plasma renin activity > 10 ng/L/hr or 150% above baseline; the test is an excellent screen to assess the need for more invasive radiographic evaluation).
Imaging	US-Renal: kidneys are asymmetrical; the left kidney is 8 cm long. **[A]** Arteriography-Renal (bilateral): stenosis of the left renal artery.
Pathogenesis	Hypertension in patients with renal vascular disease is due to excessive renin release secondary to reduced renal blood flow and perfusion pressure. This usually occurs when a single branch of the renal artery is stenosed, although bilateral obstruction may be present in up to 25% of patients. **Atherosclerotic disease** is responsible for stenosis in most older patients, whereas intrinsic structural abnormalities of the arterial wall **(fibromuscular dysplasia)** is the cause in younger patients (especially women). The condition should be suspected when hypertension occurs in a previously normotensive individual < 30 or > 50 years or in a patient who has suggestive clinical features such as epigastric or renal artery bruits, atherosclerotic disease of the aorta or peripheral arteries, symptoms of hypokalemia secondary to hyperaldosteronism (muscle weakness, tetany, polyuria), or diminished renal function

15.   SECONDARY HYPERTENSION (RENAL ARTERY STENOSIS)

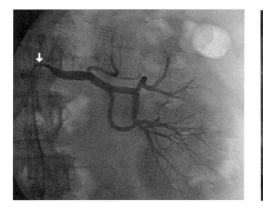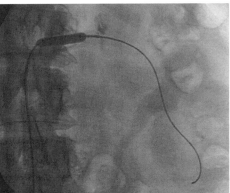

following the use of ACE inhibitors.

Epidemiology

Renal artery stenosis is a common cause of secondary hypertension, accounting for 2%–5% of cases.

Management

Treatment aimed at restoration of renal perfusion: [B] percutaneous transluminal angioplasty (PTCA) is the procedure of choice in patients with fibromuscular dysplasia and discrete stenotic lesions that do not involve the renal artery ostium. Although associated with risks, surgery remains superior to PTCA and is associated with lower restenosis rates and greater improvement or preservation of GFR. **Medical management for control of hypertension:** ACE inhibitors are the drugs of choice for unilateral renal artery stenosis (although they are contraindicated in the presence of bilateral stenosis or solitary kidney); nitroprusside and calcium channel blockers are also effective.

Complications

Renal artery stenosis is a progressive disease that may lead to indolent ischemic renal disease. This is particularly true in older patients with atherosclerotic disease, in whom narrowing can lead to complete occlusion in 10% of cases. Ischemic renal disease accounts for 15% of end-stage renal disease in patients > 50 years of age.

Associated Diseases

◘ **Coarctation of the Aorta** Congenital stenosis of the aorta usually distal to the left subclavian artery; increased incidence in patients with Turner's syndrome; presents with weak and delayed femoral pulses, upper extremity hypertension, and systolic murmur heard loudest over the back; often asymptomatic but can cause claudication on exertion; CXR shows rib notching; chest CT documents the stenosis; treat with surgical resection of the stenosis with end-to-end anastomosis; complications include severe hypertension.

■ **Pheochromocytoma** A tumor of the adrenal medulla that causes increased production of catecholamines; presents with paroxysmal attacks of headache, anxiety, and hypertension; elevated blood sugar and increased urinary vanillylmandelic acid; treat hypertensive crisis with alpha- and beta-blockers, surgical resection of tumor.

■ **Primary Aldosteronism (Conn's Syndrome)** Caused by an aldosterone-secreting adrenocortical adenoma; presents with diastolic hypertension, absence of edema, headaches, fatigue, and weakness; hypernatremia, hypokalemia, and metabolic alkalosis; elevated plasma and urinary aldosterone levels with low plasma renin activity (suggestive of primary hyperaldosteronism); ECG reveals U waves due to hypokalemia; obtain CT of abdomen to localize the adrenal adenoma; treat with surgical resection of the adenoma.

15. SECONDARY HYPERTENSION (RENAL ARTERY STENOSIS)

ID/CC	A 54-year-old stockbroker presents after suddenly fainting while eating lunch with his coworkers.
HPI	The patient has been taking **tricyclic antidepressants** for the past two years. On a few occasions over the past several months, he has also experienced heaviness in the chest on exertion (= ANGINA).
PE	VS: normal. PE: alert; neurologic and cardiac exams normal.
Labs	CBC/Lytes: normal. Calcium and glucose normal. **[A]** ECG (during episode): polymorphic ventricular tachycardia in which the axis of each successive beat changes in a characteristic "twisting of points."
Imaging	CXR: normal.
Pathogenesis	A specific type of ventricular tachycardia (VT) that is characterized by **polymorphic QRS complexes** that **change in amplitude and cycle length;** the syndrome is by definition associated with **QT prolongation.** Episodes of torsades de pointes are typically initiated by a premature ventricular beat occurring during a prolonged QT interval. The clinical effects depend on ventricular rate, the duration of the tachycardia, and the presence of underlying cardiac disease. If VT is rapid and associated with significant myocardial dysfunction or cerebrovascular disease, syncope and hypotension are likely. The diagnosis of VT can be confirmed by examining the relationship between the ECG and ventricular activity. Torsades de pointes may occur spontaneously after administration of any drug that prolongs the QT interval (e.g., tricyclic antidepressants and quinidine).
Epidemiology	N/A
Management	**Remove the precipitating cause.** When **drug-induced** (group Ia antiarrhythmic drugs, imipramine and amiodarone), **atrial or ventricular overdrive pacing** and the administration of **IV magnesium sulfate** are useful in terminating the arrhythmia. **Beta-blockers** are helpful in treating VT due to **congenital factors.**
Complications	Patients with uniform VT without heart disease have a good prognosis and a low probability of sudden death. Polymorphic VT preceded by QT prolongation (> 0.6

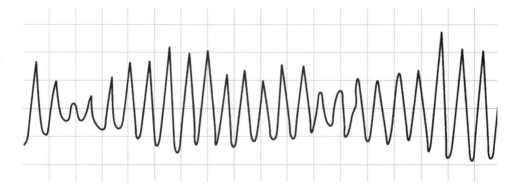

sec) may predispose patients to multiple episodes of **nonsustained VT** (< 30 sec or 10 beats) with **recurrent syncope.** However, these patients may also develop ventricular fibrillation and sudden death. **FIRST AID** **2** p. 332

FIRST AID 2 p. 332

Associated Diseases

◻ **Congenital Prolonged QT Syndrome** A genetic defect of ion channels with variable penetrance; presents with syncope in children precipitated by exertion; ECG shows long QT at baseline with ventricular tachycardia during syncopal episodes; treat with beta-blockers prophylactically; consider an implantable defibrillator for patients who have had a syncopal episode; complications include sudden cardiac death.

◻ **Ventricular Flutter** Ventricular arrhythmia with a rate of 150–300 BPM associated with ischemia or hypoxia, closely related to ventricular fibrillation; presents with acute hypotension and hemodynamic compromise or sudden death; ECG shows a regular, sinusoidal undulation without distinct P-QRS-T morphology; management is immediate defibrillation with fluid and pressor infusion to support perfusion.

ID/CC	A 32-year-old male complains of frequent **palpitations.**
HPI	He denies chest pain, syncope, or dizziness.
PE	N/A
Labs	**[A]** ECG: shortened PR interval; slurred upstroke (= DELTA WAVE); widening of QRS complex (> 0.12 sec).
Imaging	N/A
Pathogenesis	Wolff–Parkinson–White (WPW) syndrome describes patients with both preexcitation on ECG and paroxysmal tachycardias. The typical ECG patterns result from a fusion of the activation of the ventricles over both the bypass tract and the AV nodal His–Purkinje system. The impulse is typically conducted anterograde over the normal AV system and retrograde through congenital aberrant tissue. This produces a tachycardia with a wide QRS complex. Most cases are asymptomatic with evidence of preexcitation on a screening ECG. WPW syndrome can be associated with Ebstein's anomaly, mitral valve prolapse, idiopathic dilated cardiomyopathy, or hypertrophic cardiomyopathy.
Epidemiology	WPW syndrome is the most common type of ventricular preexcitation.
Management	Although surgical ablation of bypass tracts is possible and offers a permanent cure, **radiofrequency catheter ablation** of bypass tracts is safer and more cost-effective. Pharmacologic therapies are targeted at one or more components of the reentrant circuit. **Beta-blockers** or **calcium channel** antagonists increase the refractoriness of the AV node and slow conduction; **quinidine** and **flecainide** produce similar effects in the bypass tract. **IV lidocaine or procainamide** (the drugs of choice) will slow the ventricular response in severe tachycardia. If hemodynamically unstable, give DC countershock.
Complications	Atrial fibrillation occurs commonly; rarely ventricular arrhythmia may occur. Early recurrence of preexcitation may occur after a successful catheter ablation. Late recurrence is uncommon; sudden death is rare.
Associated Diseases	N/A

17. **WOLFF–PARKINSON–WHITE SYNDROME**

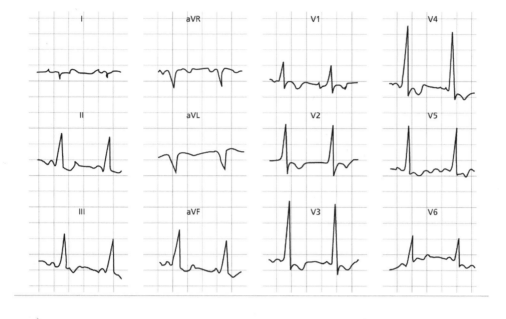

WOLFF–PARKINSON–WHITE SYNDROME

ID/CC	A 30-year-old male complains of increasing **weakness** and **fatigue** of two years' duration.
HPI	He also states that he has been feeling depressed with episodes of dizziness. He reports significant anorexia and weight loss over the past year with nearly constant **nausea.** His wife has noticed that he has become excessively irritable and restless.
PE	VS: hypotension (BP 80/50). PE: **diffuse dark-brown hyperpigmentation** noted, especially about the elbows and skin creases; oral mucosa reveals bluish-black hyperpigmented patches.
Labs	CBC: normocytic anemia; eosinophilia. ACTH stimulation test results in a subnormal rise in cortisol. Lytes: **hyperkalemia;** hyponatremia; hypercalcemia. ABGs: mild metabolic acidosis. Hypoglycemia; high ACTH levels after cosyntropin administration suggest adrenal dysfunction.
Imaging	CXR: normal (to check for tuberculosis).
Pathogenesis	Primary adrenal insufficiency, or Addison's disease, has two main origins: **granulomatous infections** such as TB and histoplasmosis (responsible for a minority of cases in the U.S.) and, more commonly, an **autoimmune disorder** in which lymphocytic and plasma cell invasion of the adrenal glands is accompanied by antiadrenal antibodies in the plasma. This condition may occur alone or with hypothyroidism secondary to Hashimoto's thyroiditis. Adrenal insufficiency can also present as part of a hereditary disorder marked by progressive myelin degeneration in the brain (adrenoleukodystrophy) or the spinal cord (adrenomyelodystrophy). Infiltration of the adrenals by opportunistic pathogens (e.g., CMV) and by Kaposi's sarcoma can complicate AIDS. Metastasis to the adrenals and disseminated meningococcal infection (Waterhouse–Friderichsen syndrome) are other causes of Addison's; drugs such as ketoconazole and etomidate may also cause adrenal insufficiency. In contrast to primary adrenal insufficiency, **secondary adrenal insufficiency** (hypothalamic or pituitary insufficiency, therapeutic use of corticosteroids) **is characterized by low levels of ACTH.**
Epidemiology	Primary adrenocortical insufficiency is relatively rare,

may occur at any age, and affects both sexes equally; because of the increasing therapeutic use of steroids, secondary adrenal insufficiency is now relatively common.

Management Monitor by watching for weight gain or hypokalemia. Increase the **steroid** dosage in periods of increased stress. Addisonian crisis (hypotension, hypoglycemia, hyperkalemia) requires IV hydrocortisone, IV glucose, and aggressive IV hydration. Hydrocortisone must be given before thyroxine when hypothyroidism and Addison's disease coexist (= SCHMIDT'S SYNDROME) to prevent exacerbation of adrenal insufficiency by thyroid hormone.

Complications Addisonian crisis.

Associated Diseases ◻ **Meningococcemia** Systemically disseminated infection with *Neisseria meningitidis;* more commonly seen in those with terminal complement component (C5–C8) deficiency; presents with sudden fever, chills, severe headache, meningeal signs, and petechial rash; hypoglycemia, hyperkalemia, and hyponatremia; gram-negative diplococci in blood, possibly in CSF; gross pathology reveals bilateral adrenal hemorrhage; treat with penicillin G, rifampin for close contacts; complications include fulminant adrenal infarction; also called Waterhouse–Friderichsen syndrome.

ID/CC	A 40-year-old female presents with **generalized muscle weakness** and **easy bruising.**
HPI	She also reports significant **weight gain** and **purplish marks** over her abdomen. The patient has been amenorrheic for the past four months and also complains of depression and inability to sleep adequately.
PE	VS: mild hypertension (BP 150/90). PE: acne; hirsutism; **[A]** "moon facies"; **[B]** another case with **central obesity** and peripheral wasting; **purple striae** on abdomen; **[C]** "buffalo hump"; **proximal muscle weakness** present.
Labs	Mildly elevated glucose. Lytes: hypokalemia; hypernatremia. Serum cortisol level high; elevated 24-hour urinary free cortisol test suggests Cushing's syndrome; partial cortisol suppression by high-dose dexamethasone test is consistent with pituitary ACTH excess (= CUSHING'S DISEASE).
Imaging	MR-Head (with contrast): microadenoma in the pituitary. CT-Abdomen: bilateral adrenal hyperplasia. CT-Abdomen: another case with left adrenal adenoma. CT of the chest and/or abdomen is required if ectopic ACTH syndrome is suspected and the source of ACTH is unknown.
Pathogenesis	Cushing's **disease** is caused by increased production of ACTH by a **pituitary adenoma,** resulting in bilateral adrenal hyperplasia and excessive cortisol. Cushing's **syndrome** is caused by a heterogeneous group of disorders that lead to excess cortisol either through ectopic ACTH production (small cell lung cancer) or through primary adrenal disorders (adrenocortical adenoma, nodular hyperplasia).
Epidemiology	Cushing's disease is most common in women of reproductive age. Endogenous Cushing's syndrome is rare.
Management	**Transsphenoidal microadenomectomy** is the treatment of choice; if pituitary imaging has identified a microadenoma, cure rates are excellent. Surgical removal is the treatment of choice for ectopic ACTH-producing tumors. Pharmacologic treatment of Cushing's syndrome (aminoglutethimide, mitotane, metyrapone) is limited to the control of extreme manifestations before

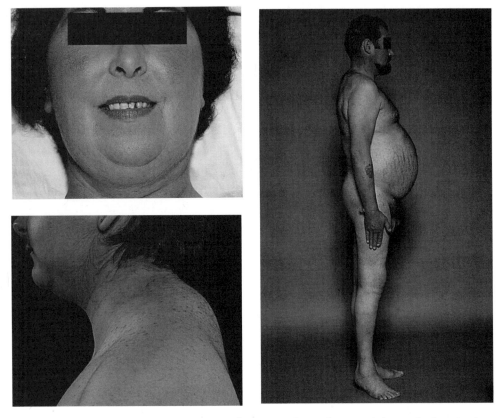

surgery, supplementation of a partial remission induced by pituitary irradiation, or inoperable patients.

Complications　　**Nelson's syndrome** develops in 10%–40% of patients after bilateral adrenalectomy. The syndrome is characterized by dramatic hyperpigmentation and by the development of a chromophobe tumor of the pituitary gland. Diabetes, infection, osteoporosis, thromboembolism, peripheral vascular disease, and ischemic heart disease may result from Cushing's syndrome.

Associated Diseases　　N/A

ID/CC	A **20-year-old white male** presents with **lethargy** that has worsened over the past 24 hours.
HPI	The patient's parents state that their son has complained of **increased thirst, frequent urination, and weight loss** (despite increased appetite) over the past several weeks. They add that he complained of **abdominal pain** today and had one episode of **emesis**.
PE	VS: no fever; normal BP; **elevated RR** (RR 25). PE: **thin and lethargic;** oriented ×3; dry mucous membranes and poor skin turgor; **fruity smell on breath** (due to ketones); **rapid, deep breathing** (= KUSSMAUL'S RESPIRATION); abdomen soft, diffusely tender to palpation, and nondistended.
Labs	Lytes: **hyponatremia** (133 mEq/L); hyperkalemia (5.8 mEq/L); hyperchloremia (115 mEq/L); **decreased bicarbonate** (6 mEq/L). Elevated BUN and creatinine; **elevated glucose** (550 mg/dL). ABGs: **acidemia** (pH 7.15). UA: **ketonuria and glucosuria**.
Imaging	N/A.
Pathogenesis	Type 1 diabetes mellitus (or insulin-dependent diabetes mellitus) is characterized by inadequate pancreatic insulin production leading to hyperglycemia and its attendant complications. Persistent hyperglycemia causes many of the chronic conditions associated with type 1 diabetes mellitus (DM) as a result of nonenzymatic glycosylation, protein deposition, and the conversion of glucose to sorbitol. Although the precise etiology of type 1 DM is unknown, it is known to be **associated with HLA-DR3 and DR4 and with autoantibodies to pancreatic islet-cell antigens.**
Epidemiology	Type 1 DM appears in 0.2%–0.5% of the population, occurs more commonly in whites, and usually presents prior to age 25. While < 10% of first-degree relatives of the proband are affected, the **concordance rate is approximately 50% with identical twins.**
Management	**Tightly regulated glucose** levels decrease the incidence and progression of complications. Patients should receive dietary **education,** regular glucose monitoring, and periodic HbA1C monitoring. Control is achieved with exogenous insulin injections or insulin pump infusions.

DIABETES MELLITUS - TYPE 1 (IDDM)

Complications	Acutely, patients may develop **diabetic ketoacidosis or hypoglycemic coma.** Long-term hyperglycemia predisposes to **diabetic nephropathy, neuropathy, retinopathy, vascular disease** (peripheral disease and CAD), nonhealing wounds, and chronic infections.
Associated Diseases	☐ **Hemochromatosis** Parenchymal accumulation of iron leading to impaired function of organs such as the heart, pancreas, liver, pituitary, and testes; the primary form (autosomal-recessive, linked to the HLA-A locus on chromosome 6) is due to dysregulated and increased intestinal iron absorption; secondary iron overload (as in thalassemia) is due to the dual effect of increased intestinal absorption and multiple blood transfusions; alcoholism is a predisposing factor (alcohol increases intestinal absorption of iron); presents with bronze skin pigmentation, diabetes mellitus, arthropathy (pseudogout), chronic liver disease, cardiac dysfunction (dilated cardiomyopathy, cardiac arrhythmias, cardiac failure) and hypogonadotropic hypogonadism; elevated serum iron, transferrin, and ferritin; elevated serum glucose; glycosuria; liver biopsy reveals evidence of chronic liver disease and markedly increased iron concentration; treat iron overload with regular phlebotomy; screen family members for disease.

☐ **Maturity-Onset Diabetes of Youth** A genetic defect in hexokinase enzyme resulting in decreased binding affinity for glucose such that elevated glucose levels are necessary to stimulate insulin release; affects non-obese teenagers; presents with asymptomatic elevations in blood glucose; treat with oral hyperglycemic agents.

☐ **Diabetic Ketoacidosis** Increased anion gap acidosis, more common in type 1 diabetes mellitus but also seen in type 2; follows infection and physical or mental stress; presents with confusion, abdominal pain, dehydration, and fruity breath smell; increased anion gap acidosis and hyperglycemia; treat with insulin and IV fluids, replete potassium, continue insulin until anion gap closes.

ID/CC	A 25-year-old male is brought to the emergency room in a **comatose state.**
HPI	He has been diagnosed with **insulin-dependent diabetes mellitus (IDDM)** and has been receiving insulin for six years. His parents report three similar incidents in the past.
PE	VS: tachycardia (HR 110). PE: comatose and moderately dehydrated; Kussmaul breathing noted.
Labs	Lytes: potassium initially normal (hydration and correction of acidosis invariably lower serum levels, unmasking profound total body depletion); hyponatremia. Serum glucose elevated. ABGs: anion gap acidosis. Elevated levels of **ketone bodies** (acetoacetate, beta-hydroxybutyrate, acetone) in urine and serum.
Imaging	N/A
Pathogenesis	The two cardinal features of diabetic ketoacidosis (DKA)—acidosis and hyperglycemia—are caused by the combined effects of severe insulin deficiency and excessive secretion of counterregulatory hormones that interact synergistically to potentiate the effects of insulin loss. These changes mobilize the delivery of substrates from muscle (amino acids, lactate, pyruvate) and adipose tissue (free fatty acids, glycerol) to the liver, where they are actively converted to glucose (via gluconeogenesis) or ketone bodies (beta-hydroxybutyrate, acetoacetate) and are ultimately released into the circulation at rates greater than the capacity of tissues to utilize them; the net result is **hyperglycemia** (> 300 mg%), increased anion gap metabolic **acidosis** (pH < 7.35), and an osmotic diuresis that leads to marked **dehydration.**
Epidemiology	DKA may herald the onset of type 1 IDDM but occurs most often in previously diagnosed diabetic patients as a result of intercurrent illness or inadequate insulin administration.
Management	**IV insulin; ample IV fluids** to compensate for dehydration; replete potassium and phosphate; sodium bicarbonate may be given to combat severe acidemia. Search for and treat underlying causes (e.g., infection). Administer dextrose once blood glucose is < 300 mg/dL. Complications of treatment are avoidable with

close monitoring but include fluid overload, cerebral edema, hypo- or hyperkalemia, and hypoglycemia. ICU admission is often required.

Complications

Impaired cardiac and respiratory function secondary to acidemia may reduce ventricular threshold to fibrillation. **Mortality** remains at 5%–15%.

Associated Diseases

◻ **Alcoholic Ketoacidosis** Increased anion gap acidosis; distinguish from diabetic ketoacidosis by hypoglycemia; seen in malnourished alcoholics; presents with altered mental status, nausea, and vomiting; anion gap metabolic acidosis; treat with IV fluids, thiamine; correct electrolyte abnormalities.

◻ **Nonketotic Hyperosmotic Coma** A hyperosmolar, hyperglycemic nonketotic coma occurring mainly in NIDDM patients; may be precipitated by physical stress; presents with severe volume depletion, stupor, tachycardia, dehydration, and confusion; markedly increased blood glucose, increased serum and urine osmolality, and glycosuria with no ketonuria; treat with aggressive IV fluid infusion, insulin, potassium, and phosphate as needed.

ID/CC	A 44-year-old female complains of a **rash on her face, abdomen, distal extremities, and perineum** (= MIGRATORY NECROLYTIC ERYTHEMA).
HPI	The patient frequently drinks large amounts of fluid, urinates often, including twice during the night, and eats voraciously (= POLYDIPSIA, POLYURIA, AND POLYPHAGIA OF DIABETES MELLITUS). Nevertheless, she acknowledges a **weight loss** of approximately 25 kg in the last year. She also states that she frequently feels lethargic and tires easily (secondary to anemia).
PE	VS: normal. PE: **rash appears erythematous, raised, and scaly** with presence of bullae and crusting; scleral icterus (secondary to hepatic metastases); **glossitis; dystrophic nails; thinning hair.**
Labs	CBC: low hematocrit (29). Glucose elevated; abnormal glucose tolerance test; **fasting plasma glucagon elevated** (> 1,000 pg/mL); total cholesterol low. LFTs: normal.
Imaging	[A] CT-Abdomen: lobulated mass (1) in the tail of the pancreas with extension into the superior mesenteric vein; solitary, metastatic lesion (2) in the right lobe of the liver.
Pathogenesis	Glucagonomas are **malignant pancreatic (alpha-2) islet cell tumors that primarily secrete glucagon** as well as other peptides, such as gastrin, insulin, somatostatin, and pancreatic polypeptide (at lower levels). They are characterized by the presence of diabetes mellitus, necrolytic migratory erythema, anemia, and weight loss. These tumors may also present in the context of MEN type I (= WERMER'S SYNDROME).
Epidemiology	These **rare** tumors are generally **solitary and slow-growing** and **present with metastatic disease, usually to the liver or bone.**
Management	**Operative resection** is curative in one-third of patients. Even if eradication is not possible, surgical debulking prolongs survival and provides effective palliation. Chemotherapeutic regimens and hepatic infusions are of little benefit.
Complications	Liver and bone metastases.
Associated Diseases	N/A

GLUCAGONOMA

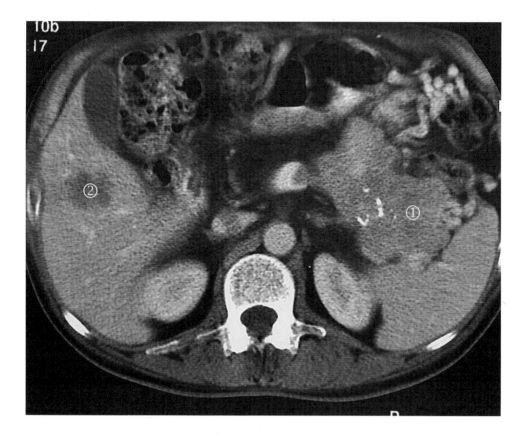

GLUCAGONOMA

ID/CC	A **45-year-old woman** presents with **generalized swelling of the neck** that has progressively worsened over the past two years.
HPI	She also has a history of chronic **constipation, cold intolerance,** skin coarseness, edema, headaches, arthralgias, **hoarseness,** and **fatigue.**
PE	VS: **bradycardia.** PE: coarse, dry skin; nonpitting **pedal edema;** midline goiter moves with deglutition; goiter rubbery with enlarged pyramidal lobe; no cervical lymphadenopathy noted.
Labs	Depressed T3 and T4; elevated TSH; high anti-thyroid peroxidase (TPO) antibody titers; high anti-thyroglobulin antibody titers. FNA: lymphocytic infiltration of gland tissue.
Imaging	N/A
Pathogenesis	Demonstration of elevated **antithyroid antibodies** in Hashimoto's thyroiditis underscores the autoimmune basis of its etiology. Inflammation may initially produce hyperthyroidism, with follicles secreting preformed thyroid hormone. Patients may then have an intervening period of euthyroidism before the disease progresses. As the inflammatory process progressively destroys thyroid tissue, compensatory hyperplasia may be unable to produce adequate thyroid hormone, and partial or severe hypothyroidism results. The presence of copious lymphocytes is a hallmark of the disease that distinguishes it from other forms of autoimmune thyroiditis.
Epidemiology	Hashimoto's thyroiditis is the most common cause of goitrous hypothyroidism in adults and children; almost all cases of primary hypothyroidism in adults are secondary to Hashimoto's thyroiditis. It is three times **more common in women** and is most frequently diagnosed between the third and fifth decades of life. A genetic propensity for the disease is demonstrated by an increased familial incidence and an association with MHC antigens such as HLA-B8.
Management	**Thyroxine** replacement is used to suppress the goiter or to correct hypothyroidism; this is continued indefinitely.
Complications	Pregnant women with high antibody titers are at high

risk for **miscarriage.** Hashimoto's commonly coexists with other autoimmune diseases, including pernicious anemia, Sjögren's syndrome, SLE, adrenal insufficiency, and diabetes mellitus.

Associated Diseases

◘ **De Quervain's Thyroiditis** A subacute inflammatory thyroiditis; idiopathic or caused by viral infections, initially causing hyperthyroidism due to leakage of thyroid hormone from inflamed gland; presents with fever, sore throat, pain over the thyroid, and jaw pain, all worsening with side-to-side motion of the head; elevated free T4, high ESR, and markedly diminished radioiodine uptake; treat with NSAIDs or corticosteroids for refractory disease until normalization of free T4 and radioactive iodine uptake; condition is often self-limiting but may progress to hypothyroidism due to gland damage.

◘ **Graves' Disease** Hyperthyroidism caused by autoantibodies activating the TSH receptor; seen in young to middle-aged women; presents with symptoms of thyrotoxicosis (weight loss despite increased appetite, fatigue, insomnia, heat intolerance, tachycardia, diarrhea, and excessive anxiety), a diffuse vascular goiter, pretibial myxedema, and exophthalmos; elevated T3 and T4; TSH is low; positive thyroid-stimulating immunoglobulins; treatment is thyroid ablation with methimazole or propylthiouracil, radioactive iodine, or surgery; propranolol for symptomatic relief; complications include atrial fibrillation and thyroid storm, which can be fatal.

◘ **Multinodular Goiter** Idiopathic autonomously functioning thyroid nodules; presents with heat intolerance, insomnia, fatigue, weight loss, increased appetite, brisk reflexes, tachycardia, palpitations, and multiple nodules palpable in gland; low TSH; increased radioiodine uptake in focal areas of thyroid with suppression of uptake in the rest of the gland; treat with radioiodine ablation or surgical excision of nodules.

ID/CC	A **55-year-old woman** complains of **nausea, vomiting, constipation, and abdominal pain.**
HPI	The patient states that she has not wanted to eat (= ANOREXIA), has lost approximately 10 pounds in the past two months, and frequently feels **fatigued, weak, and depressed.** She adds that she passed a **kidney stone** approximately one month ago.
PE	VS: normal. PE: alert and oriented ×3; hypoactive bowel sounds.
Labs	Lytes: **elevated calcium** (12.5 mg/dL); low phosphate (2.0 mg/dL); elevated chloride. **PTH elevated.** UA: **hypercalciuria.** ECG: **short QT interval.**
Imaging	XR-Skull: tiny "punched-out" lesions creating a "salt-and-pepper" appearance.
Pathogenesis	Primary hyperparathyroidism is characterized by hypercalcemia and hypophosphatemia secondary to increased PTH secretion. The causes of primary hyperparathyroidism include single or multiple parathyroid adenomas (most common cause) and hereditary hyperparathyroidism (as may be seen in association with MEN syndromes).
Epidemiology	**Ninety percent** of cases of **hypercalcemia** arise as a **result of hyperparathyroidism** or **malignancy.** Primary hyperparathyroidism is more prevalent in **middle-aged and elderly women.**
Management	**IV hydration** followed by **furosemide diuresis** to acutely lower serum calcium. Parathyroidectomy is the definitive treatment; commonly one of the resected parathyroid glands is implanted in the forearm for future use if the patient develops hypoparathyroidism. **Bisphosphonates** such as etidronate or pamidronate are used while awaiting **parathyroidectomy. Avoid thiazide diuretics.** Estrogen replacement may be offered to postmenopausal women.
Complications	**Cardiac arrhythmias** may arise with calcium levels > 12 mg/dL. Above 13 mg/dL, **metastatic calcification** (especially when phosphate is concomitantly elevated) and **renal insufficiency** may result. Above 15 mg/dL, patients are at risk for **coma and cardiac arrest.** Other complications include GI disease (pancreatitis and peptic

ulcer disease), renal disease (nephrolithiasis and nephrocalcinosis), and skeletal complications (pseudogout and osteitis fibrosa cystica).

Associated Diseases   N/A

ID/CC	A 47-year-old woman presents **following a thyroidectomy** complaining of **painful cramps and spasms in her hands** (= TETANY).
HPI	She also states that she has noticed **tingling of her hands, face, and feet** (= PARESTHESIAS). She denies any history of **bone pain** or **seizures.**
PE	VS: normal. PE: alert and oriented; tapping over facial nerve anterior to ear causes local muscle twitching (= POSITIVE CHVOSTEK'S SIGN); tetanic carpal spasm following inflation of sphygmomanometer on arm (= POSITIVE TROUSSEAU'S SIGN); 4/5 muscle strength in extremities; normal two-point and sharp/dull discrimination.
Labs	Lytes: **low calcium** (7.0 mg/dL); **elevated phosphate** (5.5 mg/dL); normal magnesium. **PTH low.** ECG: **prolonged QT interval.**
Imaging	N/A
Pathogenesis	Hypoparathyroidism is most commonly caused by parathyroid damage (due to thyroid, parathyroid, or neck surgery). Other causes include radiation-induced damage; infiltration with iron (hemochromatosis), copper (Wilson's disease), or tumor metastasis; autoimmune or familial factors; hypo- or hypermagnesemia; and DiGeorge's syndrome (congenital absence of parathyroid and thymus glands).
Epidemiology	Most commonly due to accidental damage during neck surgery; commonly occurs transiently after thyroid surgery.
Management	**Calcium gluconate** by slow IV push for acutely symptomatic patients. For long-term therapy, administer **vitamin D** and **calcium.**
Complications	Laryngeal stridor, seizures, calcification of basal ganglia leading to parkinsonian signs and symptoms, and optic lens calcification leading to cataracts.
Associated Diseases	N/A

HYPOPARATHYROIDISM

ID/CC	A 50-year-old **woman** complains of increasing **weakness, mental slowness,** and a progressive **increase in weight** despite a reduced appetite.
HPI	She also complains of wrist pain radiating to her hands as well as chronic **constipation, cold intolerance,** an increasingly husky voice (due to myxedema around vocal cords), decreased auditory acuity, and **menorrhagia.** A few years ago, she underwent a surgical thyroidectomy for Graves' disease.
PE	VS: bradycardia (HR 56). PE: expressionless face; **rough, dry skin;** brittle hair; carotenemia; scar from previous **thyroidectomy** seen; Tinel's sign and Phalen's maneuver positive (median nerve compression/carpal tunnel syndrome); delayed relaxation of DTRs.
Labs	CBC: normocytic, normochromic anemia. Low total serum T3 and T4; TSH elevated. Lytes: hyponatremia (due to SIADH). ECG: bradycardia; low voltage complexes.
Imaging	CXR: enlarged heart shadow. Echo: pericardial effusion.
Pathogenesis	The most frequent causes of hypothyroidism are **chronic Hashimoto's thyroiditis** and **ablative therapy** for hyperthyroidism. A less common cause is **neck irradiation** for cancers such as lymphoma. **Amiodarone** can cause hypothyroidism as well as hyperthyroidism; neither effect requires preexisting thyroid disease. The presence of immunoglobulins that bind to the TSH receptor but that do not stimulate thyroid function can also lead to thyroid deficiency. Finally, hypothalamic or pituitary deficiency can cause secondary hypothyroidism, but this mechanism accounts for < 5% of cases.
Epidemiology	The incidence of hypothyroidism varies somewhat with **geographic area.** In areas with adequate iodine supply (e.g., the U.S.), only 0.82%–1.0% of the population is hypothyroid; in **iodine-deficient areas,** however, the incidence is **10- to 20-fold higher.** The prevalence of hypothyroidism is **greater in females** than in males (5–15 vs. 1 in 100).
Management	Synthetic **thyroid hormone replacement;** treat until TSH normalizes and patient is symptom free. CAD is a

relative contraindication to thyroxine administration and should be addressed prior to the initiation of therapy.

Complications   Myxedema coma. Hyperlipidemia and ischemic heart disease are associated with long-standing hypothyroidism.

Associated Diseases   ◘ **Myxedema Coma** A complication of severe hypothyroidism, usually precipitated by infection; common in elderly females; presents with hypothermia, hypoventilation, hypotension; hyponatremia, hypoxia, and hypercapnia; treat with levothyroxine; intubate if necessary.

ID/CC	A **56-year-old** male is brought to the ER in a state of **confusion**.
HPI	His sister states that he had previously been complaining of intermittent episodes of **slurred speech, headaches, and visual disturbances.** These episodes usually **occurred after periods of fasting** and were **alleviated by eating.**
PE	VS: tachycardia. PE: oriented to person but not place or time; **tremulous, diaphoretic,** and **pale;** lungs clear to auscultation bilaterally.
Labs	Low glucose (23 mg/dL); **serum insulin elevated; proinsulin elevated; C-peptide elevated** (rules out surreptitious insulin administration); cortisol normal (rules out hypothalamic-pituitary-adrenal axis abnormality).
Imaging	[A] MR-Abdomen: the inversion recovery technique shows an enhancing mass in the tail of the pancreas. [B] MR-Abdomen: before gadolinium is given, a low-signal mass is seen in the tail. [C] The mass is seen to enhance after administration of gadolinium. [D] Angio: another case shows a round, vascular lesion in the pancreatic head.
Pathogenesis	Insulinomas are **beta-cell neoplasms** that are located primarily in the pancreas. Increased insulin production can lead to **Whipple's triad,** which consists of **(1) symptoms of hypoglycemia; (2) fasting hypoglycemia; and (3) relief of symptoms with administration of IV glucose and restoration of normoglycemia.** The hypoglycemia subsequently induces catecholamine release and consequent symptoms.
Epidemiology	Insulinomas are **rare** tumors that generally appear in the **fifth to seventh decade as single, benign adenomas.** Ten percent are multiple and 10% are malignant (spread to local lymph nodes and liver). They may also present in the context of MEN type I.
Management	Treat acutely with **IV or oral glucose.** Definitive therapy involves **surgical removal** of the adenoma or partial pancreatectomy. If surgery is not possible, patients should receive diazoxide or octreotide (inhibits insulin release) and streptozocin and doxorubicin

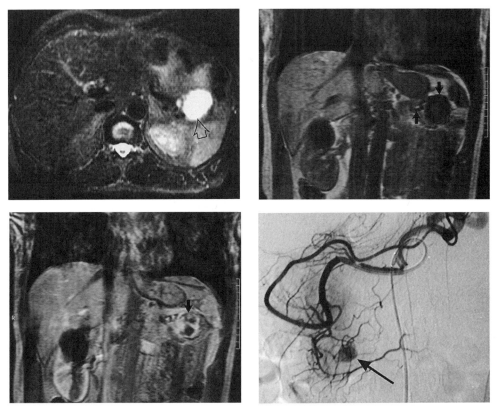

(chemotherapy combination of choice for insulinoma).

Complications   Hypoglycemic episodes may result in trauma, brain injury, coma, or death.

Associated Diseases   ◻ **Glycogen Storage Diseases** Genetic defects of enzymes in the glycogen synthetic or degradative pathways; present with organomegaly involving the liver, heart, kidney, or muscle; hypoglycemia and exercise intolerance; enzyme assay of tissue reveals deficiency; treat with frequent carbohydrate-rich meals to ameliorate symptoms; complications include lactic acidosis and growth retardation.

ID/CC	A **70-year-old** man with a prior history of **non-insulin-dependent** diabetes mellitus (NIDDM), CAD, hypertension, and glaucoma presents to the ER with complaints of increasing lethargy over the past week.
HPI	He also complains of **urinary frequency** and **persistent thirst.** He has become increasingly lethargic and **confused.**
PE	VS: supine BP normal, P 80; standing BP 98/65, P 102 (= ORTHOSTATIC HYPOTENSION). PE: lethargic, uncommunicative, oriented to person only, and in mild distress; skin pale, cool, and tented; pallor; lungs clear.
Labs	**Elevated glucose** (> 600 mg/dL); **hyperosmolality.** ABGs: **pH normal** (no acidosis); serum HCO_3 normal; normal anion gap (9–14 mEq/L). Lytes: hyponatremia (120–125 mEq/L). Elevated BUN (101 mg/dL) with normal creatinine (= PRERENAL AZOTEMIA).
Imaging	N/A
Pathogenesis	Nonketotic hyperosmolar syndrome occurs in patients with type 2 diabetes mellitus **(NIDDM)** who have a partial or relative insulin deficiency; in it, there is a decrease in peripheral utilization of glucose that induces glucagon secretion, which in turn stimulates hepatic gluconeogenesis. As a result of massive hyperglycemia, glucose excretion in urine increases, producing a strong osmotic diuresis. This produces significant plasma volume contraction, dehydration, and reduced renal perfusion. Renal hypoperfusion results in decreased urinary glucose loss and even higher blood glucose concentrations. Consequently, a severely hyperosmolar state develops, resulting in mental confusion and eventually coma. Since the basal requirement of insulin is not compromised, ketosis does not occur.
Epidemiology	The **second most common form of hyperglycemic coma;** usually found in patients with either mild or occult diabetes (more than half of patients were previously undiagnosed with NIDDM). **Middle-aged and elderly patients** are most likely to be affected. Predisposing factors include renal insufficiency and CHF, both of which are associated with a poorer

prognosis.

Management

Fluid replacement with isotonic saline should be initiated immediately if the patient is hypovolemic. In all other cases, hypotonic saline (0.45%) should be used because the body fluids of patients are often severely hyperosmolar. Nearly 4–6 L of fluid may be required in the first 8–10 hours. Careful monitoring of sodium and H_2O replacement is important. Replace **potassium** and administer **insulin.** Once blood glucose drops to 250 mg/dL, fluid replacement should include 5% dextrose infusion that is titrated to maintain glycemic levels of 250–300 mg/dL.

Complications

The overall mortality of nonketotic hyperglycemic hyperosmolar coma is > 10 times that of diabetic ketoacidosis primarily because of its higher incidence in older patients with significant comorbidity, as well as the delay in recognition (and treatment) of this syndrome.

Associated Diseases

◻ **Diabetic Ketoacidosis** Increased anion gap acidosis, more common in type 1 diabetes mellitus but also seen in type 2; follows infection and physical or mental stress; presents with confusion, abdominal pain, dehydration, and fruity breath smell; increased anion gap acidosis and hyperglycemia; treat with insulin and IV fluids, replete potassium, continue insulin until anion gap closes.

NONKETOTIC HYPERGLYCEMIC COMA

ID/CC	A 54-year-old man from Siberia complains of **pelvic weakness** that he experiences when he rises to a standing position from a seated position.
HPI	The patient is a refugee from a Siberian prison who sought political asylum in the United States. His symptoms are associated with bone pain and **tenderness** in the pelvic region but are also present to a lesser extent in his spine. The patient also reports that he experienced significant weight loss secondary to **poor nutrition** during the last two years of his imprisonment. He was locked up in a dark cell with other prisoners prior to his escape.
PE	VS: normal. PE: thin and poorly nourished; localized **tenderness in pelvic girdle and spine** with moderate decrease in proximal lower extremity motor strength.
Labs	CBC/Lytes: normal. **Low serum calcium (< 4.2 mg/dL); low serum phosphate; increased alkaline phosphatase; low 25-hydroxyvitamin D; low urine calcium.**
Imaging	[A] XR-Spine: decreased bone density and partial central collapse of all vertebral bodies. [B] XR-Femur: another case shows a horizontal lucency with sclerotic margins (= LOOSER'S ZONE) in the cortex of the medial femur.
Pathogenesis	Osteomalacia is characterized by defective mineralization of organic bone matrix that may result from inadequate dietary intake or malabsorption of vitamin D (as in chronic pancreatitis with exocrine insufficiency), acquired or inherited disorders of vitamin D metabolism (anticonvulsant therapy, renal failure), chronic acidosis (renal tubular acidosis, acetazolamide ingestion), renal tubular defects that produce hypophosphatemia (Fanconi's syndrome), and aluminum toxicity.
Epidemiology	Rare in the U.S. as a result of adequate dietary intake; common in underdeveloped countries owing to dietary deficiency and poverty. In developed countries, it is seen with food fads or eating disorders (e.g., anorexia nervosa). Inadequate sun exposure may be seen in the elderly. Malabsorption may be seen in patients with a history of pancreatic or other GI disease, whereas defects in vitamin D metabolism may be seen in patients with

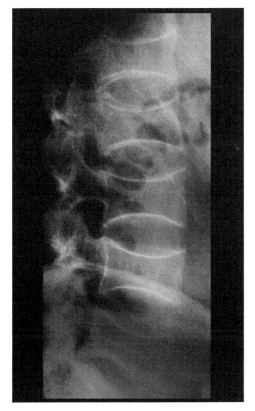 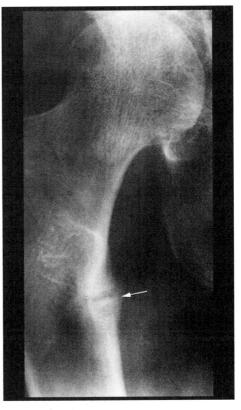

liver or renal disease.

Management Correct the underlying cause; supplement vitamin D. Supplement phosphate and calcium as needed. Radiologic evidence of recovery is seen at 1–6 months.

Complications Bone pain and tenderness may develop quickly, particularly within the spine, ribs, pelvis, and lower extremities. Proximal muscle weakness is also common, especially in the lower extremities. Fractures may occur with minimal trauma.

Associated Diseases ◘ **Rickets** Vitamin D deficiency most commonly due to lack of sun exposure or nutritional deficiency in children; presents with poor skull mineralization (= CRANIOTABES), costochondral thickening (= RACHITIC ROSARY), kyphoscoliosis, varus deformity of legs, and tetany; hypocalcemia; radiologic alterations are most evident at the epiphyseal growth plate (particularly of the radius and ulna), which is increased in thickness, cupped, and hazy at the metaphyseal border owing to decreased calcification and inadequate mineralization; treat with vitamin D, calcium, and phosphate supplements.

ID/CC	An 81-year-old woman presents with **altered mental status, irritability,** and **confusion** over the past day.
HPI	Her family notes that she has had occasional episodes of previously unreported **intermittent hemoptysis** and chest pain over the past three months. She has **smoked** two packs of cigarettes per day for 60 years.
PE	VS: normal. PE: disoriented; lung, cardiac, and abdominal exams normal.
Labs	CBC: normal. Lytes: **hyponatremia** (128 mEq/L). **Low serum osmolality; elevated urine sodium** (> 20 mmol/L); **concentrated urine** (increased urine osmolality); **detectable plasma ADH** (normally unmeasurable); cytology of sputum demonstrates malignant cells consistent with **small cell carcinoma.**
Imaging	CXR: hilar masses with mediastinal widening.
Pathogenesis	SIADH characteristically produces dilutional hyponatremia without edema. It may result from ectopic production of ADH from neoplasms (small cell lung carcinoma, duodenal carcinoma, pancreatic carcinoma) and tuberculous lung parenchyma; from increased ADH release from the neurohypophysis following **intracranial lesions** (meningitis, trauma, encephalitis, SAH); or from drug-induced stimulation of ADH release (vincristine, chlorpropamide, carbamazepine) or potentiation of ADH effects (chlorpropamide, NSAIDs).
Epidemiology	N/A
Management	Correct hyponatremia with water restriction, sodium replacement, and loop diuretics. Correct rapidly to 120–125 mmol/L and then slowly correct over 24–48 hours to a normal range in order to prevent the development of **central pontine myelinolysis.** Restrict fluid intake or administer saline depending on the patient's volume status. Causes of SIADH should be identified and corrected. Demeclocycline is the most potent inhibitor of ADH action and may be useful for chronic SIADH (untreatable malignancy or CNS disease).
Complications	Complications include confusion, seizures, or coma. Prognosis depends on the primary etiology.
Associated Diseases	◻ **Addison's Disease** Adrenocortical failure commonly

caused by autoimmune disease, infection, or acute infarction; presents with hypotension, weakness, nausea/vomiting, and hyperpigmentation; presentation can be subacute or catastrophic; hyponatremia, hyperkalemia, and metabolic acidosis (due to lack of aldosterone production); hypoglycemia (due to lack of glucocorticoid production); failure of cortisol levels to rise following ACTH stimulation is diagnostic; management is lifelong replacement of hormones via hydrocortisone and fludrocortisone; doses of hormones must be increased during infections or acute stressors; complications include electrolyte imbalances and hemodynamic collapse.

◘ **Hypothyroidism** Decreased thyroid activity most commonly caused by Hashimoto's thyroiditis; may also be caused by surgery and radioactive iodine treatment; presents with weakness, lethargy, cold intolerance, weight gain, hoarseness, depression, constipation, menorrhagia, delayed recovery phase of DTRs, and nonpitting edema (= MYXEDEMA); may see pericardial effusion; low T3 and T4 and elevated TSH; hyponatremia (due to SIADH); elevated serum cholesterol and triglycerides; elevated CK and anti-TPO/anti-microsomal antibodies (in Hashimoto's thyroiditis); treat with levothyroxine

ID/CC	A 10-year-old boy complains of headache, **malaise,** nausea, vomiting, **loss of appetite,** and **fever** with chills for the past week.
HPI	He also complains of passing **dark-colored urine.**
PE	VS: fever (39.2 C); mild tachycardia (HR 105); normal BP. PE: **icterus; tender hepatomegaly.**
Labs	LFTs: **AST and ALT markedly increased;** mild elevation in alkaline phosphatase and bilirubin. **Anti-HAV IgM present.**
Imaging	N/A
Pathogenesis	The causative agent is hepatitis A virus (HAV), an RNA virus of the picornavirus family; it is transmitted by the **fecal-oral route** and produces an acute viral hepatitis. Unlike hepatitis B and C virus infections, chronic hepatitis A infection does not occur. Anti-HAV IgG confers immunity.
Epidemiology	HAV transmission is enhanced by poor personal hygiene, contaminated food, and certain sexual practices. **No HAV carrier state has been identified,** and inapparent subclinical infection maintains the virus in nature.
Management	**No specific treatment. Rest** during the acute phase. Hospitalization may be required for severely ill patients. Alcohol, high fat intake, and drugs that produce adverse effects on the liver or require liver metabolism should be avoided. Give hepatitis A and B vaccine for travelers to endemic areas. Hepatitis B vaccine is recommended for health care workers and children < 12 years who did not receive the series as infants.
Complications	Relapse occurs only rarely but remains self-limited (hepatitis A). Rare complications include myocarditis, cholestatic hepatitis, pancreatitis, aplastic anemia, atypical pneumonia, transverse myelitis, and peripheral neuropathy. Fulminant hepatitis is very rare; risk factors include increasing age and chronic liver disease.
Associated Diseases	◘ **Chronic Active Hepatitis** Persistent inflammation with necrosis of the liver lasting > 6 months, caused by viral infections, hepatotoxic drugs, autoimmune disease, Wilson's disease, or alpha-1-antitrypsin deficiency; may

also be of unknown etiology; presents with anorexia, malaise, jaundice, and hepatomegaly; elevated aminotransferases and alkaline phosphatase; serology for viral markers (HBV, HCV), autoantibodies for autoimmune hepatitis (ANA, anti-LKM antibody, anti-SMA); serum and urinary copper levels for Wilson's disease; serum electrophoresis for alpha-1-antitrypsin deficiency; liver biopsy reveals evidence of bridging and piecemeal necrosis; treat viral infections with interferon with or without ribavirin or lamivudine; complications include progression to cirrhosis, hepatic encephalopathy, and hepatocellular carcinoma.

ID/CC	A 59-year-old **male** with a history of **alcoholism** presents with **persistent upper abdominal** (= EPIGASTRIC) **pain that radiates to the back.**
HPI	The pain was **initially episodic** but is now **constant,** is not relieved by antacids, and is worsened by the ingestion of alcohol or fatty foods. The patient denies nausea or vomiting (vs. acute pancreatitis) but states that he frequently has **foul-smelling, loose, bulky, greasy stool** (= STEATORRHEA). He adds that he has lost 20 pounds over the past year.
PE	VS: low-grade fever (38.2 C). PE: cachectic; jaundiced (secondary to edema and fibrosis at the head of the pancreas causing common bile duct obstruction); mild epigastric tenderness without rebound or rigidity.
Labs	CBC/PBS: decreased hematocrit; megaloblastic anemia (30). Lytes: hypocalcemia. Serum **vitamin B_{12} levels low; impaired glucose tolerance; low serum cholesterol;** amylase and lipase normal; **elevated serum trypsinogen levels; reduced pancreatic enzyme secretion** on stimulation; stool exam reveals **increased fecal fat.**
Imaging	[A] KUB: multiple **calcifications** in the distribution of the pancreas. [B] CT-Abdomen: punctate calcifications within the pancreas. [C] US-Abdomen: **"chain of lakes"** deformity of the pancreatic duct caused by many strictures with intervening areas of dilation; splenic vein (1). [D] ERCP: a dilated and irregular pancreatic duct.
Pathogenesis	Chronic pancreatitis is characterized by **extensive pancreatic fibrosis,** clinically presenting with pain, malabsorption, or repeated episodes of acute inflammation in a previously damaged pancreas. Causes include **alcoholism** (the most common cause of pancreatic exocrine insufficiency in adults in the U.S.), **cystic fibrosis** (the most common cause in children), or causes of **acute pancreatitis** (which lead to recurrent episodes of pancreatic inflammation, as seen in chronic relapsing pancreatitis); it may also be idiopathic.
Epidemiology	Alcohol-induced pancreatitis is more common in **males,** with an age of onset between 40 and 49 years. Most cases in children are secondary to cystic fibrosis.
Management	Therapy is directed toward **eliminating the underlying**

CHRONIC PANCREATITIS

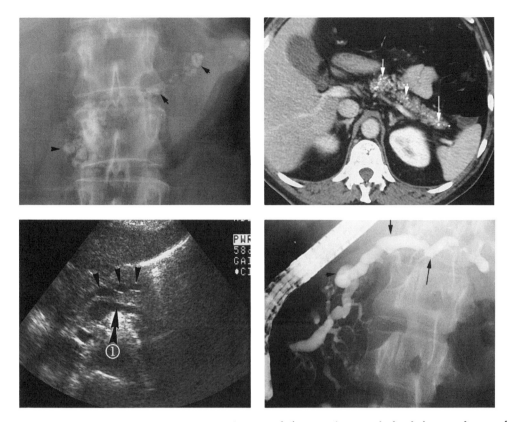

cause, treating malabsorption, minimizing pain, and delaying disease progression. Consequently, patients should be encouraged to abstain from alcohol; give NSAIDs or narcotics (long-term use should be avoided) for pain, vitamin supplements (fat-soluble vitamins and vitamin B_{12}), and pancreatic enzymes with antacids for malabsorption (enzymes are inactivated below a pH of 4). Patients who develop diabetes may require insulin. In cases of intractable pain, surgery should be considered.

Complications
Complications include diabetes mellitus, pancreatic exocrine insufficiency, pancreatic cancer, pancreatic pseudocyst or abscess (in acute exacerbations), common bile duct or duodenal obstruction, splenic vein thrombosis, ascites, and pleural effusion. Narcotic dependence may become an issue. **FIRST AID 2** p. 145

Associated Diseases
◻ Acute Pancreatitis Most commonly caused by alcoholism and gallstones; other causes include hypertriglyceridemia and hypercalcemia; may also be hereditary, idiopathic, or drug induced (azathioprine, didanosine, furosemide, estrogens); presents with excruciating abdominal pain radiating to the back,

nausea, vomiting, and tachycardia; hypoxemia, hypocalcemia, hyperglycemia, leukocytosis, elevated amylase, and elevated lipase; CT shows pancreatic edema; treat with IV fluids, pressors as needed, narcotics for analgesia; make patient NPO until symptoms resolve; complications include hemodynamic compromise, systemic inflammatory response syndrome, and pancreatic pseudocyst.

CHRONIC PANCREATITIS

ID/CC	A **24-year-old Jewish male** complains of persistent **nonbloody diarrhea.**
HPI	The patient states that he has experienced fecal incontinence with small amounts of stool (perianal fistula). He has also had **colicky lower abdominal pain, weight loss, anorexia,** and periodic **joint pain.**
PE	VS: fever (38.4 C); normal HR, RR, and BP. PE: thin and **pale** (secondary to anemia); temporal wasting; abdomen soft with **right lower quadrant tenderness and fullness;** no hepatosplenomegaly; orifice posterior to anus expresses stool (= PERIANAL FISTULA).
Labs	CBC: normal WBC; decreased hematocrit (28). PBS: normochromic, normocytic RBCs. ESR elevated. LFTs: normal. Stool negative for ova and parasites; colonoscopy shows grossly inflamed colon with serpiginous ulcers separated by areas of normal mucosa (= SKIP LESIONS); colonic biopsy reveals **noncaseating granuloma formation.**
Imaging	**[A]** BE: numerous aphthoid ulcers are seen as well as loss of haustral markings in this section of the transverse colon. **[B]** BE: the mucosal **"cobblestone"** pattern is seen in this patient. **[C]** SBFT: another case reveals two distinct areas of stricture formation (1) as well as a pseudodiverticulum (2). **[D]** BE: another case shows multiple fistulae between the rectum and vagina.
Pathogenesis	The etiology of Crohn's disease (regional enteritis) is unknown; however, several genetic (based on twin and sibling studies), infectious, and immunologic (based on identifiable T-cell abnormalities) theories have been advanced. It is characterized by **transmural inflammation that may extend from the mouth to the anus.** Gross lesions appear as **serpiginous or linear ulcerations** with areas of intervening normal mucosa and **cobblestoning** with **stricture and fistula formation.** Histologically, they are characteristically seen as **noncaseating granulomas with crypt distortion and lymphocytic infiltration.**
Epidemiology	Crohn's arises in approximately 0.1% of the population and in approximately 17% of individuals with an affected first-degree relative. The disease presents most commonly in the **third decade,** but a second peak in

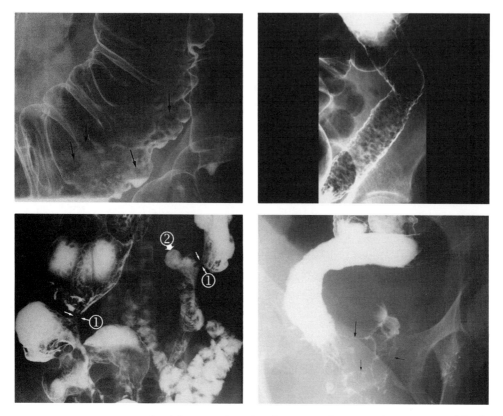

incidence arises in those aged 50–65. It occurs with the highest frequency in **Jewish men** (relative risk six times that of normal).

Management

Suppress disease activity with **corticosteroids** and **sulfasalazine** (or other 5-ASA derivatives). **Immunosuppressive agents** (methotrexate and/or azathioprine) may be used for refractory disease. Patients may require vitamin B_{12} injections and increased levels of calcium and vitamin D. Surgery, including **stricturoplasty** and/or **resection,** is indicated in cases of recurrent obstruction, enterocutaneous fistulas, and disease refractory to medical therapy.

Complications

Intestinal obstruction, perforated viscus, erythema nodosum, pyoderma gangrenosum, episcleritis, uveitis, peripheral arthritis, fistulas, and renal oxalate stones. Crohn's disease is not associated with as significant an increase in cancer risk as ulcerative colitis, although patients are at increased risk when compared to normal patients. **FIRST AID 2** p. 142

Associated Diseases

◻ **Pyoderma Gangrenosum** A large necrotic erosion commonly appearing on the shins, with heaped-up borders; idiopathic but related to ulcerative colitis and seronegative spondyloarthropathies; presents with an acute-onset dark nodule that grows in size and then ulcerates; treat the underlying disease.

◼ **Primary Sclerosing Cholangitis** Idiopathic fibrosis of bile ducts; associated with inflammatory bowel disease; presents in young males with insidious onset of jaundice and progressively worsening systemic pruritus; elevated alkaline phosphatase, hyperbilirubinemia, and transaminitis; ERCP demonstrates diffuse, multifocal biliary strictures; treat with ursodiol to reduce bile acid levels; only liver transplantation can prevent death; complications include hepatic cirrhosis with portal hypertension.

◼ **Uveitis** Inflammation of the iris, ciliary body, and choroid due to infection or systemic inflammation (e.g., inflammatory bowel disease); presents with acute, painful red eye, no loss of vision, miotic pupil, and circumcorneal ciliary congestion; slit-lamp exam shows cells and flare in the anterior chamber; treat with steroids, cycloplegics and antibiotics if an infectious etiology is suspected.

◼ **Ulcerative Colitis** An inflammatory bowel disease limited to the mucosa and submucosa of the colon and rectum; presents with crampy abdominal pain, tenesmus, and passage of blood and mucus in stool; colonoscopy shows mucosal erythema, granularity, inflammatory polyps, and continuous lesions; treat with sulfasalazine, corticosteroids, surgery; complications include toxic megacolon, extraintestinal manifestations (erythema nodosum, pyoderma gangrenosum, seronegative spondyloarthropathy, uveitis, episcleritis), and a significantly increased risk of colon cancer.

◼ **Primary Biliary Cirrhosis** An inflammatory disorder affecting the extra- and intrahepatic bile ducts; most commonly found in middle-aged women; associated with inflammatory bowel disease; presents with pruritus, jaundice, gallstones, xanthelasma, and progressive hepatic cirrhosis; conjugated hyperbilirubinemia, hyperlipidemia, and elevated anti-mitochondrial antibody titers (> 1:40); treat with cholestyramine for symptomatic relief; consider liver transplant.

CROHN'S DISEASE

ID/CC	A **71-year-old** female presents to the emergency room with painless **bright red blood per rectum** (= HEMATOCHEZIA).
HPI	She states that she frequently feels **constipated** and strains on defecation. She reports that her diet is **low in fiber.**
PE	VS: no fever; tachycardia (HR 120); tachypnea (RR 20); normal BP. PE: alert and oriented; **pallor;** cool extremities; 2-sec capillary refill; regular rate and rhythm; abdomen soft, nontender, and nondistended; positive bowel sounds; **bright red blood in rectal vault.**
Labs	CBC: normal WBC; depressed hemoglobin (8.0) and hematocrit (24); normal platelets. Coagulation studies normal; nasogastric tube negative for blood or bile.
Imaging	**[A]** BE: multiple diverticula are seen as outpouchings of the sigmoid colon. **[B]** BE: another case reveals a pericolic abscess (barium is seen outside the bowel lumen); the serrated appearance of the bowel wall is due to muscle hypertrophy. **[C]** BE: another case demonstrates a colonic stricture surrounded on both sides by many diverticula.
Pathogenesis	Occur as a result of **high intraluminal pressure** distributed throughout a narrow lumen (such as the sigmoid colon), causing **herniations that lack a muscularis** (= FALSE DIVERTICULA). These typically **arise at sites where arterioles traverse the colonic wall** and are prone to bleeding. These outpouchings may also become obstructed, permitting growth of bacteria and consequent inflammation (= DIVERTICULITIS).
Epidemiology	Colonic diverticula occur in approximately 33% of individuals > 40 years and in **> 50% of individuals > 70 years.** Risk factors include a **low-fiber diet** (and therefore low stool weight) and living in a developed country.
Management	**High-fiber diet** and **transfusion for significant blood loss.** In cases of severe hemorrhage, mesenteric angiography is diagnostic and therapeutic (with intra-arterial embolization). In cases of recurrent diverticulitis, patients should consider sigmoidectomy with a primary colorectal anastomosis.

DIVERTICULOSIS

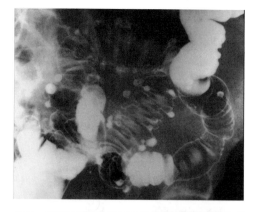
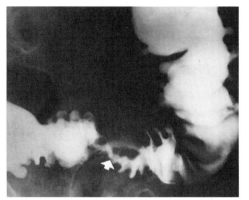
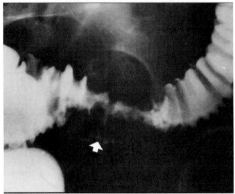

Complications	**Exsanguinating hemorrhage** is associated with untreated diverticular bleeds. Diverticulitis may lead to **abscess formation, peritonitis, fistula formation, and perforation.**
Associated Diseases	◘ **Diverticulitis** Inflammation of the diverticula; presents with fever, nausea, vomiting, acute abdominal pain, and cramping; can be diffuse or localized to the left lower quadrant; leukocytosis; abdominal CT may show diverticula with mesenteric fat stranding indicating inflammation; treat with IV fluids; make NPO until episode passes; Bactrim and metronidazole; complications include perforation and peritonitis.

◘ **Ischemic Colitis** Most commonly caused by atherosclerosis of the celiac axis and mesenteric artery; also caused by embolism, arteritis, and venous thrombosis; presents with extreme abdominal pain 30 minutes after eating and with nausea, vomiting, bloody diarrhea, markedly distended abdomen, rebound tenderness, and heme-positive stool; treat with emergent |

laparotomy to prevent complete infarction, perforation, peritonitis, and sepsis.

◘ **Pseudomembranous Colitis** Pseudomembrane formation in the colon due to overgrowth of *Clostridium difficile;* results from antibiotic use, commonly clindamycin or ampicillin; presents with watery diarrhea with pus and mucus; presence of toxin in stool; treat with metronidazole or vancomycin.

ID/CC	A 50-year-old woman complains of **heartburn** and **burping** exacerbated by eating.
HPI	She states that her symptoms are **worsened when she lies down.** She has a 40-pack-year **smoking** history and is currently being treated with **diltiazem** for hypertension.
PE	VS: mild hypertension (BP 146/88). PE: epigastrium tender on deep palpation.
Labs	Endoscopically obtained mucosal biopsies (from 5 cm above the lower esophageal sphincter) show changes of chronic esophagitis.
Imaging	**[A]** Barium Swallow: another case with hiatus hernia and refluxed barium into hiatus.
Pathogenesis	Chronic esophagitis is most often the result of toxic damage to the esophageal lining secondary to gastroesophageal reflux.
Epidemiology	Risk factors for reflux include hiatal hernia, incompetent lower esophageal sphincter (LES), obesity, pregnancy, and scleroderma.
Management	Treatment focuses on **decreasing acid production** (proton pump inhibitors, H$_2$ receptor antagonists), **improving LES tone,** and increasing gastric motility **(metoclopramide).** Intervention should include **smoking cessation,** education on proper use of antacids, elevation of the patient's head during sleep, **dietary restriction** (alcohol, mints, chocolate, fat, and caffeine), and weight loss. Medications that decrease LES tone (e.g., calcium channel blockers) should be avoided. Consider **surgery** (fundoplication, repair of hiatal hernia) for those who have not responded to medical therapy and lifestyle modification. Regular endoscopic surveillance should be conducted to rule out Barrett's esophagus and adenocarcinoma.
Complications	Esophageal stricture, chronic aspiration, asthma, bleeding, and **Barrett's esophagus** (a risk factor for adenocarcinoma).
Associated Diseases	**◻ Achalasia** An idiopathic disorder of esophageal peristalsis and inadequate relaxation of the lower esophageal sphincter (LES); presents with dysphagia,

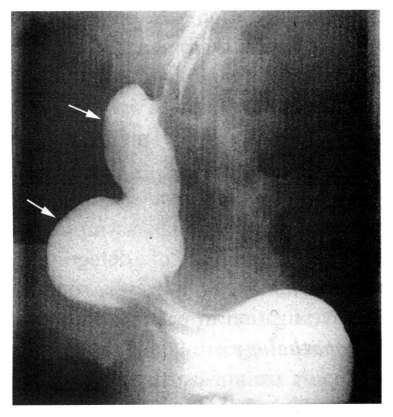

regurgitation, and retrosternal chest pain; UGI reveals "rat-tail" narrowing of the esophagus at the lower sphincter; treat mild cases with medical measures such as oral nitrates, calcium channel blockers, or endoscopic injection of botulinum toxin into the LES; other cases require endoscopic balloon dilatation or extramucosal myotomy of the LES.

◻ **Barrett's Esophagus** Premalignant metaplasia of the distal esophageal squamous epithelium to a columnar epithelium in response to prolonged acid reflux; presents with retrosternal burning, belching, and water brash; endoscopy reveals epithelial metaplasia; treat with cisapride and proton pump inhibitors; complications include a markedly elevated risk of esophageal adenocarcinoma.

◻ **Acute Hemorrhagic Gastritis** Caused by ingestion of corrosive substances, corticosteroids, alcohol, or aspirin, or secondary to severe systemic stress; presents with nausea, vomiting, epigastric pain, coffee-ground emesis,

GASTROESOPHAGEAL REFLUX DISEASE

tachycardia, and hypotension; anemia and occult blood in stool; UGI reveals erosions and fold thickening; EGD reveals petechial hemorrhages and small mucosal ulcerations; treat with antacids, IV fluids, and transfusion as needed; complications include hemodynamic collapse.

◘ **Chronic Atrophic Gastritis** Atrophy secondary to chronic gastritis of any etiology, commonly autoimmune affecting the fundus or related to *H. pylori* infection affecting the antrum and body of the stomach; presents with megaloblastic anemia in autoimmune disease (pernicious anemia) or dyspepsia with *H. pylori* disease; gastric biopsy reveals atrophy; plasma B_{12} level low in pernicious anemia; serum antibodies against *H. pylori;* treat with B_{12} replacement for autoimmune disease and omeprazole, metronidazole, and clarithromycin for *H. pylori* disease; complications of *H. pylori* disease include increased risk of gastric carcinoma.

35.   GASTROESOPHAGEAL REFLUX
            DISEASE

ID/CC	A **50-year-old white male** presents with progressive **jaundice,** a peculiar skin rash, and palpitations; he also complains of generalized **fatigue** and **muscle weakness.**
HPI	The jaundice has progressively worsened over the past two years. On directed questioning, the patient notes a decrease in libido and complains of pain in the left knee for the past three months. He has been diagnosed with **hyperglycemia** (= BRONZE DIABETES) and dilated cardiomyopathy with atrial fibrillation. He does not smoke or drink alcohol.
PE	VS: irregularly irregular pulse. PE: **bronze discoloration** seen diffusely, especially in sun-exposed areas; icterus; loss of pubic and axillary hair; testicular atrophy; gynecomastia; spider nevi noted on chest and upper back; **liver enlarged** 5 cm below right costal margin; liver firm, nontender, and nonpulsatile; left knee swollen and tender.
Labs	Elevated blood glucose; decreased serum testosterone and gonadotropins; increased serum iron; decreased TIBC; transferrin saturation > 80%; serum ferritin elevated (> 1000 ug/L; best screening method). LFTs: elevated bilirubin; elevated AST and ALT; mildly elevated alkaline phosphatase. **Liver biopsy** shows high levels of stainable iron. ECG: atrial fibrillation (iron deposition in the heart with disruption of conduction pathways).
Imaging	[A] XR-Knee: characteristic meniscal cartilage calcification (chondrocalcinosis). US-Abdomen: liver with diffuse parenchymal infiltration suggestive of hepatitis. Echo: dilated cardiomyopathy.
Pathogenesis	Hemochromatosis is characterized by excessive deposition of iron in parenchymal cells; it is transmitted by an autosomal-recessive gene located on chromosome 6 and is caused by an **inappropriate increase** in **iron absorption** from the GI tract (normally, the amount of iron accumulated inversely affects GI mucosal absorption of both heme and non-heme iron). As iron overload progresses, iron that is ordinarily stored in the cells of the reticuloendothelial system is **deposited in the liver, joints, gonads, pancreas, heart,** and **skin.** This pattern of deposition reflects the density of transferrin receptors in these tissues.

HEMOCHROMATOSIS

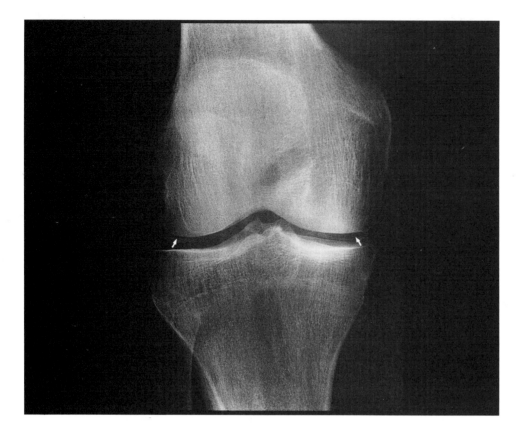

Epidemiology Hemochromatosis is the most common single gene disorder of people of Caucasian descent. Most patients have HLA-A6 antigens. Despite an equal frequency of homozygosity, **males express clinical symptoms 10 times more often than females;** this may be due to regular menstrual and childbirth-associated blood loss in women.

Management **Regular phlebotomy;** symptomatic management of joint and cardiac disease. Continue treatment until serum studies normalize or anemia develops. **Screen family** members. Cirrhosis may require transplantation.

Complications **Heart failure, cirrhosis,** and **hepatocellular carcinoma** occur in end-stage disease.

Associated Diseases ◘ **Alcoholic Liver Disease** A continuum of early adipose infiltration in the liver leading to hepatitis and finally cirrhosis, portal hypertension, and hepatic encephalopathy; presents with jaundice, ascites, hepatosplenomegaly, spider angiomata, and palmar erythema; AST is elevated more than ALT; liver biopsy demonstrates Mallory bodies with cirrhotic changes; treat with alcohol cessation; fatty liver is reversible; recurrent hepatitis induces cirrhotic changes; once cirrhosis occurs, only liver transplantation can treat the disease; complications include development of hepatocellular carcinoma.

◻ **Wilson's Disease** An autosomal-recessive disorder of copper metabolism with increased intestinal copper absorption and diminished excretion in bile with resultant deposition, primarily in the brain and liver; presents with neuropsychiatric disturbances, intellectual impairment, choreiform movements, Kayser–Fleischer rings in the cornea, and chronic liver disease; decreased serum ceruloplasmin; increased concentration of copper in biopsied liver tissue, and increased urinary excretion of copper; treat with penicillamine; complications include hepatic cirrhosis.

ID/CC	A 47-year-old male complains of **lack of appetite** (= ANOREXIA), **weakness,** malaise, and **increasing abdominal girth** (= ASCITES).
HPI	He also complains of marked **weight loss, impotence,** tea-colored urine, and passage of black, tarry, foul-smelling stools (= MELENA). He was hospitalized a few weeks ago for treatment of **hematemesis.** He is a **heavy drinker.**
PE	VS: tachycardia (HR 105). PE: **muscle wasting;** mild **jaundice;** pallor; loss of axillary, chest, and pubic hair; enlargement of parotid glands; **palmar erythema; gynecomastia; spider nevi** in abdominal skin; caput medusae; **liver markedly enlarged** with a hard and nodular consistency (liver is small in end-stage cirrhosis); **splenomegaly;** positive fluid wave sign (due to ascites); testicular atrophy; pedal edema.
Labs	CBC: **macrocytic anemia; thrombocytopenia.** Elevated PT. LFTs: AST/ALT ratio > 2:1 (typical of alcoholic hepatic damage); elevated alkaline phosphatase; elevated GGT; elevated **bilirubin.** High blood ammonia; low serum albumin; liver biopsy (CT-guided) reveals destruction of normal architecture with **regenerating nodules** and **fibrotic** changes; UGI endoscopy reveals presence of esophageal varices.
Imaging	UGI: filling defects in **"string of beads"** pattern (esophageal varices). **[A]** CT-Abdomen: the liver is seen to be shrunken and irregular with a regenerative nodule (1) in the caudate lobe; splenomegaly (2) with multiple perisplenic varices is also seen. **[B]** CT-Abdomen: a different case shows not only splenomegaly but also dilatation of the left renal vein (1) and inferior vena cava (both the result of portosystemic shunting). **[C]** CT-Abdomen: a different case demonstrates massive ascites (3); note the liver (1) and inferior vena cava (2).
Pathogenesis	Cirrhosis is pathologically characterized by diffuse, irreversible, widespread hepatic parenchymal fibrosis in association with the formation of regenerative nodules. It is caused by **alcohol,** viruses (hepatitis B and C), biliary cirrhosis, extrahepatic biliary obstruction, hemochromatosis, alpha-1-antiprotease deficiency, cystic fibrosis, schistosomiasis, and Wilson's disease.

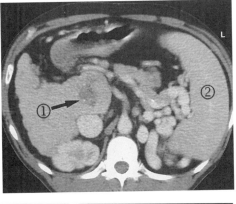
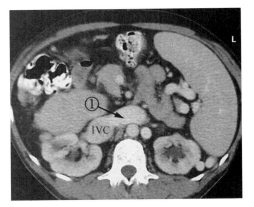
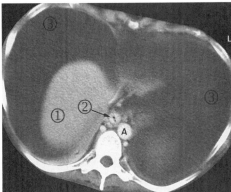

Histologically, it is divided into two variants: **macronodular** (= POSTNECROTIC; usually associated with viral hepatitis) and **micronodular** (= LAËNNEC'S; typically associated with alcohol).

Epidemiology Cirrhosis is the third leading cause of death in men in the fifth decade of life and the eleventh leading cause of death in the U.S. It also predisposes patients to hepatocellular carcinoma. Thirty percent of patients with cirrhosis die within one year of diagnosis.

Management **Cessation of alcohol use** is key. Hemorrhagic complications are managed with vitamin K and fresh frozen plasma. Ascites is managed with large-volume paracentesis, **salt/protein restriction,** and **diuretics.** Encephalopathy due to liver failure responds to decreased protein intake and **neomycin** and **lactulose** (to decrease serum ammonia). Spontaneous bacterial peritonitis is treated with IV antibiotics. Variceal bleeding may require **sclerotherapy,** transjugular intrahepatic portosystemic shunt (TIPS), or **surgical anastomosis.**

Complications Encephalopathy, variceal bleeding, portal vein thrombosis, hypersplenism, liver failure, nutritional deficiencies, coagulopathy, and spontaneous peritonitis.

FIRST AID 2 p. 63

Associated Diseases N/A

ID/CC	A 49-year-old **male** presents with **anorexia**, nausea, and **jaundice**.
HPI	He also reports pain in his right upper quadrant and darkening of his urine. He has been a **heavy drinker** for the past five years and recently went on a week-long alcohol binge.
PE	VS: normal. PE: jaundice; tender hepatomegaly.
Labs	CBC: macrocytic anemia (due to folate deficiency); thrombocytopenia. Elevated PT. LFTs: AST and ALT elevated with > 2:1 ratio; elevated bilirubin and alkaline phosphatase. Liver biopsy (CT-guided) reveals hepatocyte necrosis, Mallory bodies, infiltration of neutrophils, and perivenular fibrosis; UGI (endoscopy) reveals no esophageal varices but shows superficial gastric erosions with small petechiae.
Imaging	N/A
Pathogenesis	The **amount and duration of alcohol consumption** are directly related to the development of alcoholic hepatitis. Initially, consumption of alcohol leads to the deposition of fat within hepatocytes. This leads to neutrophilic infiltration, hepatocyte **necrosis**, and collagen deposition in perivenular spaces and eventually to **cirrhosis**.
Epidemiology	Alcoholism affects > 10 million Americans. Alcohol-induced hepatitis accounts for approximately 38% of all cases of chronic hepatitis. Risk factors for alcoholism include male gender, family history, regular drinking prior to age 16, Native American heritage, psychiatric illness, and antisocial personality.
Management	Therapy is initially directed toward cessation of alcohol abuse and **management of complications** of the illness, such as variceal bleeding. Treat alcohol withdrawal; give vitamin supplements (including B_{12}, thiamine, and folate).
Complications	Complications include **cirrhosis**, which in turn predisposes patients to **hepatocellular carcinoma**, variceal bleeding, encephalopathy, and ultimately death. Nutritional deficiencies may produce **Wernicke's encephalopathy** (confusion, ataxia, ophthalmoplegia) resulting from thiamine deficiency. Long-term thiamine deficiency results in **Wernicke–Korsakoff syndrome** (a

chronic amnestic disorder characterized by confabulation).

◘ **Alpha-1-Antitrypsin Deficiency** Variable deficiency of enzyme that inhibits trypsin, elastase, and collagenase, causing proteolytic destruction of lung and liver in variable combinations; presents with panacinar emphysema or hepatic cirrhosis; PFTs reveal FEV_1/FVC < 75%; liver biopsy shows cirrhosis; treat emphysema with home oxygen; only transplant can treat liver disease.

◘ **Hepatocellular Carcinoma** A primary liver malignancy associated with cirrhosis, most often of viral etiology; presents with jaundice, cachexia, abdominal distention, ascites, and a hard nodular liver; decreased serum albumin, prolonged PT, and markedly elevated serum alpha-fetoprotein; US and CT reveal an enhancing hepatic mass; treat with tumor embolization, chemotherapy, surgical resection if metastases are not found during workup.

◘ **Hepatorenal Syndrome** Acute renal failure associated with severe hepatic disease; presents with acute-onset oliguria in patients with sequelae of liver disease; elevated BUN and creatinine; treat with diuretics, dialysis if necessary; consider liver transplant; high mortality.

◘ **Wilson's Disease** An autosomal-recessive disorder of copper metabolism with increased intestinal copper absorption and diminished excretion in bile with resultant deposition, primarily in the brain and liver; presents with neuropsychiatric disturbances, intellectual impairment, choreiform movements, Kayser–Fleischer rings in the cornea, and chronic liver disease; decreased serum ceruloplasmin, increased concentration of copper in biopsied liver tissue, and increased urinary excretion of copper; treat with penicillamine; complications include hepatic cirrhosis.

ID/CC	A **22-year-old female** complains of **colicky abdominal pain** and **diarrhea** that occur 10 minutes after she starts eating.
HPI	She also complains of a **bloated sensation** with **lower abdominal distention** that is more marked in the **late afternoon.** She reports increasing stress secondary to job pressure.
PE	VS: normal. PE: appears well nourished; no pallor, cyanosis, or jaundice; **abdomen mildly distended, tympanic, and tender in hypogastrium;** no masses or peritoneal signs; hyperactive bowel sounds.
Labs	CBC/Lytes: normal. LFTs: normal. UA: normal. No occult blood in feces; stool ova and parasites negative; TFTs normal; sigmoidoscopy normal.
Imaging	BE: **dilatation of sigmoid colon** with no other sign.
Pathogenesis	Also called **spastic colitis** or nervous colitis, it is an idiopathic, **functional** intestinal motility disorder with a strong **relationship to stress.**
Epidemiology	Irritable bowel syndrome is one of the most common disorders seen by the primary care practitioner. The disorder shows a **female predominance,** generally starts in the late teens or early 20s, and is typically associated with a wide array of other "psychosomatic" diseases. It is a **diagnosis of exclusion** that is made once organic pathology has been ruled out and if symptoms are known to have persisted for at least 3–6 months.
Management	**Reassurance;** psychiatric counseling; **high-fiber diet** low in irritants and gas-producing foods. Diphenoxylate and atropine/loperamide (for diarrhea) or psyllium/mild laxatives (for constipation); antidepressants, anxiolytics, or prokinetic drugs.
Complications	An increased incidence of **diverticulosis** is caused by prolonged constipation. Major psychological comorbidity also results in "doctor shopping" and dependency on narcotics or benzodiazepines.
Associated Diseases	◻ **Celiac Sprue** Gluten-sensitive enteropathy in genetically susceptible hosts (associated with HLA-DR3); presents with diarrhea, flatulence, steatorrhea, bone pain (due to osteomalacia), easy bruising (due to vitamin K

deficiency), weight loss, dermatitis herpetiformis, and failure to thrive in children; iron deficiency anemia, IgA anti-gliadin antibodies, and increased fecal fat; a small intestinal biopsy showing blunted villi is characteristic; treat with gluten-free diet (free from the protein component of grains such as wheat, rye, barley and oats); complications include iron deficiency anemia and intestinal lymphoma.

◘ **Crohn's Disease** Inflammatory bowel disease; can involve any part of the GI tract, commonly the terminal ileum; presents with intermittent right lower quadrant abdominal pain, bloody diarrhea, an abdominal mass in the right iliac fossa, and perianal fistulas; colonoscopy may reveal "cobblestoning," skip lesions of inflammatory edema, fibrosis, and transmural inflammation; treat with corticosteroids and sulfasalazine; consider surgical excision of bowel segments for refractory disease; complications include uveitis, arthritis, and gallstones.

◘ **Lactase Deficiency** Deficiency of enzyme that hydrolyzes lactose into glucose and galactose; common in premature infants; develops in the majority of non-European populations during early adulthood; presents with abdominal bloating, cramps, and flatulence; treat by avoidance of lactose-rich foods, replacement of lactose enzyme.

◘ **Pseudomembranous Colitis** Pseudomembrane formation in the colon due to overgrowth of *Clostridium difficile*; results from antibiotic use, commonly clindamycin or ampicillin; presents with watery diarrhea with pus and mucus; presence of toxin in stool; treat with metronidazole or vancomycin.

◘ **Ulcerative Colitis** An inflammatory bowel disease limited to the mucosa and submucosa of the colon and rectum; presents with crampy abdominal pain, tenesmus, and passage of blood and mucus in stool; colonoscopy shows mucosal erythema, granularity, inflammatory polyps, and continuous lesions; treat with sulfasalazine, corticosteroids, surgery; complications include toxic megacolon, extraintestinal manifestations (erythema nodosum, pyoderma gangrenosum, seronegative spondyloarthropathy, uveitis, episcleritis), and a significantly increased risk of colon cancer.

ID/CC	A 42-year-old **male** business executive complains of **recurrent dyspepsia** over the past month.
HPI	The patient reports **epigastric discomfort** that he describes as gnawing, dull, achy, intermittent, episodic, and often **relieved by food.** He acknowledges a high-stress lifestyle with frequent business travel; he also **smokes** two packs of cigarettes per day and drinks an average of 1–2 martinis per day with more on weekends.
PE	VS: normal. PE: abdomen soft; mild tenderness to deep palpation in midepigastrium; no occult blood in stool.
Labs	CBC: hematocrit normal. Rapid urease breath test positive; serum *H. pylori* antibody positive; gastric mucosal biopsy reveals *H. pylori* infection; no evidence of malignancy.
Imaging	**[A]** UGI: a barium-filled ulcer crater is seen on the lesser curvature of the stomach. **[B]** UGI: a large ulcer crater is seen in the body of the stomach. **[C]** UGI: another case showing multiple ulcers in the duodenum. **[D]** UGI: scarring and stricture formation in the duodenum secondary to long-standing peptic ulcer disease is seen in another case; note the stomach (1).
Pathogenesis	Peptic ulcers represent breaks in the gastric or duodenal mucosa that arise when normal mucosal defenses are compromised or are overwhelmed by acid and pepsin. *H. pylori* (a small, microaerophilic, urease-producing, gram-negative bacillus) has a close etiologic association with virtually all (95%–100%) duodenal ulcer and most (75%–85%) gastric ulcer cases. Gastric ulcers are biopsied because up to 3%–5% of even benign-appearing lesions prove to be malignant. Nonhealing ulcers are particularly suspicious for malignancy.
Epidemiology	Peptic ulcer disease has a lifetime prevalence of approximately 10% in the U.S. adult population. Duodenal ulcers are five times more common than gastric ulcers and are typically located in the bulb or pyloric channel, while gastric ulcers are most commonly found in the antrum (60%) or the lesser curvature at the antrum-body junction (20%). Ulcers are slightly more common in men than in women (1.3:1). Duodenal ulcers tend to occur in a younger age group (35–55 years), while gastric ulcers tend to occur in an older age group (55–70

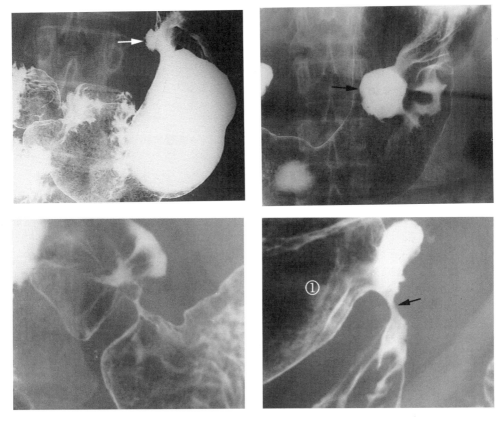

years). **Smoking** and **chronic NSAID use** are predisposing factors; alcohol, diet, and stress are also associated.

Management
Therapy is directed toward **ulcer healing and eradication of** *H. pylori*. *H. pylori*–associated ulcer disease is treated with a 10- to 14-day, **two- or three-antibiotic regimen** (ampicillin, clarithromycin, tinidazole) **combined with a proton pump inhibitor** for 4–8 weeks to promote ulcer healing. Antacids and H_2 blockers are useful adjuncts. All patients with gastric ulcers or those whose symptoms persist despite adequate therapy should undergo endoscopy with biopsy after 6–12 weeks to rule out malignancy. Patients with severe recurring ulcers should be worked up (gastrin levels) to rule out Zollinger–Ellison syndrome (gastrinoma).

Complications
Hemorrhage, perforation, gastric outlet obstruction, and gastric carcinoma.

Associated Diseases
☐ **Gastroesophageal Reflux Disease** Acid reflux from the stomach commonly seen in smokers; presents with heartburn that worsens when supine and is relieved with antacids; a small hiatal hernia may be seen on UGI; treat

with prokinetic agents (cisapride), antacids, H_2 receptor blockers, or proton pump inhibitors; patients should refrain from smoking, alcohol intake, or caffeine intake (weaken esophageal sphincter tone); complications include Barrett's esophagus (a premalignant lesion).

ID/CC	A **42-year-old woman** is hospitalized with **jaundice** and **itching.**
HPI	The patient is currently being treated for rheumatoid arthritis.
PE	VS: normal. PE: **jaundice;** scleral icterus; **hepatomegaly** and hepatic tenderness; **xanthomas** on elbows and knees.
Labs	Hypercholesterolemia (> 200 mg/dL). LFTs: **elevated alkaline phosphatase;** elevated bilirubin. **Positive antimitochondrial antibodies.**
Imaging	**[A]** ERCP: markedly decreased arborization (1) of the intrahepatic biliary tree; the extrahepatic biliary tree appears normal in this patient. Note the gallbladder (2) and endoscope (3).
Pathogenesis	Primary biliary cirrhosis is an idiopathic **autoimmune disease** characterized by the presence of **antimitochondrial antibodies** and by the destruction and loss of interlobular bile ducts, leading to **severe obstructive jaundice** and **hypercholesterolemia.** The disease progresses to hepatic cirrhosis, portal hypertension, and complications arising from these conditions.
Epidemiology	Almost all symptomatic cases occur in **women aged 35–60 years.**
Management	Treatment of hyperlipidemia may require chronic **dietary modification** and use of **lipid-lowering drugs.** Agents include resins (e.g., cholestyramine), statins (e.g., lovastatin), and niacin. Gemfibrozil is indicated if hyperlipidemia includes elevated triglycerides. In primary biliary cirrhosis, the typical treatment is ursodeoxycholic acid, which delays the progression of the disease. Currently, **liver transplant** is the only definitive therapy.
Complications	Liver failure; increased cardiovascular risk (from hypercholesterolemia).
Associated Diseases	■ **Cirrhosis** Necrosis of hepatocytes leading to hepatic fibrosis; causes include alcohol, hepatitis B and C, and hemochromatosis; presents with palmar erythema, spider angiomata (in the distribution of the superior vena cava), icterus, shrunken liver, hyperestrogenic effects

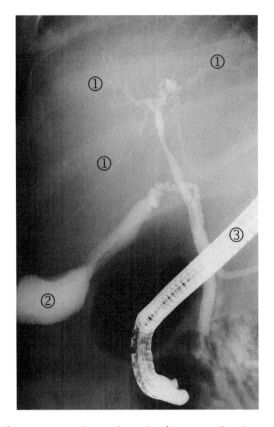

(gynecomastia and testicular atrophy in males), portal hypertension (splenomegaly, ascites, variceal bleeding), coagulopathy (due to decreased hepatic production of clotting factors), and hepatic encephalopathy (asterixis, altered mental status); hyperbilirubinemia, low serum albumin, prolonged PT, elevated liver enzymes, and high serum ammonia; treat by cessation of alcohol intake and avoidance of other hepatotoxic agents; treat portal hypertension and hepatic encephalopathy; consider liver transplant for cure.

◻ **Crohn's Disease** Inflammatory bowel disease; can involve any part of the GI tract, commonly the terminal ileum; presents with intermittent right lower quadrant abdominal pain, bloody diarrhea, an abdominal mass in the right iliac fossa, and perianal fistulas; colonoscopy may reveal "cobblestoning," skip lesions of inflammatory edema, fibrosis, and transmural inflammation; treat with corticosteroids and sulfasalazine; consider surgical excision of bowel segments for refractory disease; complications include uveitis, arthritis, and gallstones.

ID/CC	A **35-year-old female** presents with **bloody diarrhea** and associated tenesmus; she also reports significant **weight loss** and **fatigue.**
HPI	She has suffered similar episodes in the past that have been treated as bacillary dysentery. Her grandmother suffered from inflammatory bowel disease.
PE	VS: low-grade fever (38.1 C); tachycardia (HR 110); orthostatic hypotension. PE: pallor; mild tenderness in lower abdomen; heme-positive brown stool.
Labs	CBC: normochromic, normocytic anemia; mild leukocytosis (13,000). Low serum albumin; lower endoscopy shows coarse and friable mucosal surface without skip areas; rectal biopsy shows superficial inflammation with crypt abscesses; stool cultures negative; stool ova and parasites negative.
Imaging	**[A]** BE (avoid during acute phase): loss of haustral markings; narrow, foreshortened colon and loss of redundancy in the rectosigmoid region (= LEAD PIPE COLON); microulcerations.
Pathogenesis	Ulcerative colitis is primarily an inflammatory disease affecting the superficial epithelial layer of the rectum and the colon. Disease begins in the rectum and progresses proximally in a continuous fashion (no skip lesions) to involve the colon; remissions and exacerbations are common. The etiology of this disease is unknown; chronic inflammation suggests that the cause may be a regulatory alteration of mucosal immunity. **[B]** A surgically resected colonic specimen with ulceration and pseudopolyps.
Epidemiology	Inflammatory bowel disease is 2–4 times more common among **Jews** than among non-Jews and four times more common among **whites** than among nonwhites. Ten percent of patients have **family members** within two generations who also have the disease, and more than one-third know of a relative who has it. Symptomatic ulcerative colitis usually develops between 25 and 45 years of age.
Management	**Bowel rest** and IV fluids; drugs used include antidiarrheals, 5-ASA derivatives, **corticosteroids** (systemic or enemas), or immunosuppressive agents.

ULCERATIVE COLITIS

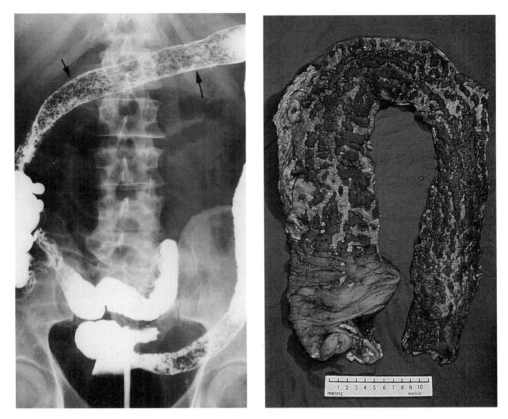

Surgery is indicated in refractory disease, toxic megacolon, colon cancer, and severe dysplasia. Perform **surveillance colonoscopy** annually after 8–10 years of disease; consider prophylactic colectomy in view of the markedly increased risk of colon cancer.

Complications

Complications include toxic megacolon, intestinal perforation, severe bleeding, and increased risk of **colon cancer.** Extraintestinal manifestations include **arthritis, erythema nodosum, pyoderma gangrenosum,** aphthous ulcers, and **iritis/uveitis.** `FIRST AID 2` p. 142

Associated Diseases

◻ **Amebiasis** Colonic infection by *Entamoeba histolytica;* presents with diarrhea with mucus, abdominal cramps, and flatulence; stool culture reveals causative protozoan.

◻ **Ischemic Colitis** Most commonly caused by atherosclerosis of the celiac axis and mesenteric artery; also caused by embolism, arteritis, and venous thrombosis; presents with extreme abdominal pain 30 minutes after eating and with nausea, vomiting, bloody diarrhea, markedly distended abdomen, rebound

ULCERATIVE COLITIS

tenderness, and heme-positive stool; treat with emergent laparotomy to prevent complete infarction, perforation, peritonitis, and sepsis.

◻ **Colorectal Cancer** Adenocarcinoma of the colon; the second most common cancer in females, third in males; shows a genetic predisposition; may be associated with a low-fiber, high-fat diet; presents with bloody stools, fatigue and weakness, diarrhea or constipation, heme-positive stool, and anemia; colonoscopy and BE reveal presence of mass; treat with partial or total colectomy; treat metastatic disease with radiotherapy and chemotherapy.

ID/CC	A **65-year-old** female complains of **palpitations.**
HPI	The patient also reports **fatigue** (due to anemia), **dysphagia** (due to oropharyngeal candidiasis secondary to neutropenia), and **easy bruising** and **epistaxis** (due to thrombocytopenia). She was recently hospitalized with **pneumonia.**
PE	VS: **fever** (38.7 C); mild tachycardia (HR 105). PE: **pallor;** numerous bruises; **petechial hemorrhages** on tonsils and skin; **[A] gum hypertrophy;** white oropharyngeal plaques; axillary **lymphadenopathy;** sternal tenderness; hepatosplenomegaly.
Labs	CBC/PBS: **anemia** (Hb 9); **low platelet count** (40,000); **leukopenia** (2,000); **[B] circulating blasts with Auer rods** (pathognomonic for leukemia). Elevated uric acid and LDH. UA: hyperuricosuria (secondary to increased cell turnover). **Bone marrow biopsy** reveals **increased proportion of blast cells** (> 30%) with prominent **staining with peroxidase and Sudan black** as well as staining for CD33 and CD13 (subtype M3/promyelocytic); cytogenetic testing reveals 15:17 translocation.
Imaging	CXR: no mediastinal mass (rules out T-cell ALL).
Pathogenesis	Acute myelogenous leukemia (AML) arises most commonly as a result of **clonal proliferation** of multipotential precursors of granulocytes, macrophages, erythrocytes, and megakaryocytes. Etiologic factors include **heredity** (chromosome aneuploidy syndromes such as Down's and Klinefelter's syndromes or diseases with excessive chromosome fragility such as Fanconi's anemia or Bloom syndrome), **radiation, chemical exposure** (e.g., benzene), and **antineoplastic drugs** (e.g., alkylating agents). Several subtypes of AML have been attributed to translocations that lead to the production of oncogenic proteins: t(8;21) in M2, t(15;17) in M3, and t(9;11) in M5. Replacement of normal marrow with leukemic marrow leads to pancytopenia and to the sequelae of the disease.
Epidemiology	Seen more commonly in individuals **> 60 years old** and in patients with **chronic myeloproliferative disorders** and **myelodysplastic syndromes.**

ACUTE MYELOGENOUS LEUKEMIA

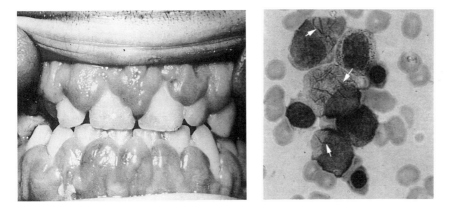

| Management | Remission may be achieved using induction **chemotherapy (cytosine arabinoside and anthracycline)** followed by intensive postremission chemotherapy or **bone marrow transplant** (allogeneic or autologous). Recurrences are effectively treated only with bone marrow transplant. Use of ATRA (all-trans retinoic acid) improves the outcome in M3 AML (as in this case). |

| Complications | Patients often develop substantial **local and disseminated infections,** bleeding complications (DIC, GI bleeding), urate nephropathy, and cerebral leukostasis. Those receiving bone marrow transplants may develop **graft-versus-host disease.** Relapse may occur. **FIRST AID 2** p. 192 |

| Associated Diseases | ☐ **Acute Lymphocytic Leukemia** The most common pediatric neoplasm; good prognosis; presents with marked weakness, pallor, bone pain, epistaxis, recurrent infections, and sternal tenderness; anemia, lymphocytosis with excess blasts, and thrombocytopenia; CALLA and TDT positive; treat with induction, consolidation, and maintenance chemotherapy; consider CNS radiation for prophylaxis against recurrence, bone marrow transplant for relapsed disease.

☐ **Myelodysplastic Syndromes** Syndromes characterized by refractory anemia and pancytopenia in which at least two cell lines are morphologically abnormal; presents with fatigue, bleeding, infection, and splenomegaly; bone marrow hyperplastic; treat with RBC transfusion, erythropoietin; consider bone marrow transplantation. |

ID/CC	A **14-year-old** female is brought to the ER because of **abdominal pain and distention, inability to evacuate and pass flatus per rectum,** nausea, and **vomiting** (intestinal obstruction).
HPI	She is a healthy girl who is fully immunized and has not traveled outside the U.S.
PE	VS: slight fever (38.3 C); tachycardia (HR 102); tachypnea (RR 22); normal BP. PE: dehydration; no jaundice; pallor; neck supple with no lymphadenopathy; **abdomen distended, tympanitic,** and tender; bowel sounds increased; no peritoneal signs; no masses; no hepatosplenomegaly; laparotomy revealed an **ileal mass** that produced an intussusception.
Labs	CBC: mild **leukocytosis;** no neutrophilia. **Elevated LDH;** tumor aspirate sent for intraoperative cytology reveals Burkitt's lymphoma cells (basophilic, nongranular nuclei; 2–5 nucleoli; eccentric, thin cytoplasm) on Romanowsky's stain (Wright or Giemsa); histopathology of mass reveals **"starry sky" pattern** (confirms diagnosis).
Imaging	CXR: normal. XR-Humerus: osteolytic bone lesion (second primary or metastasis).
Pathogenesis	A high-grade, undifferentiated B-lymphocyte **lymphoblastic lymphoma** that has two major clinical presentations. The **African type** is endemic, is associated with EBV infection, and presents as a jaw or abdominal tumor that may spread to the bone marrow. The **American** type is sporadic and has an abdominal presentation that includes ascites along with skin, bone, and peripheral node involvement.
Epidemiology	A **pediatric** disease with **a mean age of onset of seven,** it occurs mostly during the second half of the year (environmental factor?) and **more often in males.** If found in a patient > 20 years of age, it is usually a pregnant women with a breast tumor. It is the most common malignant pediatric tumor in Africa and the most rapidly growing malignant tumor in man (may double in size in 24 hours). **Predisposing** factors include **EBV** (African type), reovirus type 3, herpesvirus, **malaria** (mitogenic for B lymphocytes; causes defective cellular immunity), periodontal infections, and

BURKITT'S LYMPHOMA

chromosome 8;14 translocation.

Management   Start cyclophosphamide immediately (side effects include ovarian fibrosis, male sterility, and hemorrhagic cystitis, which may be prevented with MESNA). Combination chemotherapy consists of methotrexate, vincristine, and cytosine arabinoside with or without prednisone. Chemotherapy can cause tumor lysis syndrome, which presents with joint pains, hyperkalemia, hyperphosphatemia, hypocalcemia, and hyperuricemia. Recurrences arise within the first six months, usually in the CNS.

Complications   Metastatic and recurrent disease, bleeding, and infection.

Associated Diseases   ◻ **Hodgkin's Lymphoma** Malignancy of lymphoid tissue, linked in some patients to EBV infection; presents with generalized lymphadenopathy, hepatosplenomegaly, fever, night sweats, and weight loss, or may present with asymptomatic adenopathy; chest and abdominal CT may reveal adenopathy and hepatosplenomegaly; lymph node biopsy shows Reed–Sternberg cells (necessary but not sufficient for diagnosis); treat with radiation therapy for local disease, allowing a nearly 90% five-year survival rate; add chemotherapy for metastatic disease.

ID/CC	A **66-year-old** male presents for a routine physical.
HPI	The patient has **no complaints.**
PE	PE: pallor, **palpable axillary lymph nodes;** splenomegaly; hepatomegaly.
Labs	CBC/PBS: **anemia; thrombocytopenia; lymphocytosis** (>15,000); **[A]** **mature**, slightly smaller lymphocytes (1) and **smear cells** (2). Reduced serum immunoglobulins; **bone marrow biopsy reveals diffuse infiltration by mature lymphocytes;** lymphocyte marker analysis reveals CD19, CD20, CD21, and CD24 (= B-CELL ANTIGENS).
Imaging	CT-Abdomen: hepatosplenomegaly.
Pathogenesis	Chronic lymphocytic leukemia (CLL) is a neoplasm that usually arises from clonal proliferation of activated **B cells** (> 95%). Its etiology is unknown, but several chromosomal abnormalities, including trisomy 12, have been identified. Chromosomal abnormalities are associated with shortened survival. Patients with CLL are staged on the basis of nodal involvement and the presence of anemia or thrombocytopenia. In the international classification, **stage A** is lymphocytosis with < 3 lymph node groups; **stage B** includes involvement of > 3 lymph node groups; and **stage C** is assigned in the presence of anemia or thrombocytopenia, which may be due to bone marrow compromise, spleen involvement, or an autoimmune cause.
Epidemiology	The **most common form of adult leukemia** in the U.S., accounting for 25%–40% of all cases and increasing in frequency with age (90% occur in patients > 50). The disease is uncommon in Asian countries.
Management	Start treatment when patients are symptomatic. Stage A patients do not receive chemotherapy given that their survival is > 10 years; stage B and C patients require **chemotherapy** (alkylating agents, fludarabine, pentostatin, cladribine). **Glucocorticoids** are useful in cases of Coombs-positive hemolytic anemia, immune thrombocytopenia, and pancytopenia.
Complications	CLL may transform into a **prolymphocytic leukemia** or a **high-grade lymphoma.** Patients are also susceptible to infections (due to hypogammaglobulinemia) such as

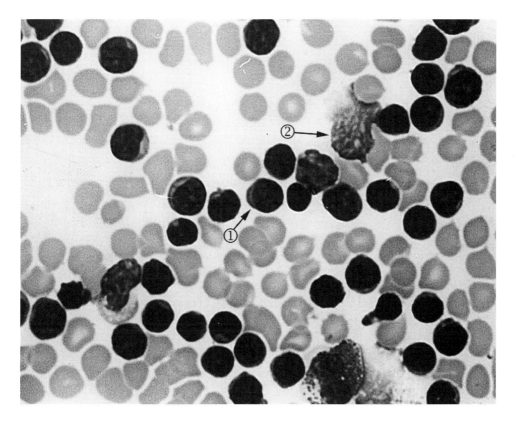

pneumococcal pneumonia and shingles as well as to hematologic derangements such as anemia, thrombocytopenia, and neutropenia. **FIRST AID 2** p. 144

Associated Diseases

◘ **Sézary Syndrome** The leukemic phase of mycosis fungoides; usually seen in middle-aged men; presents with fever, malaise, and erythematous, scaly, extremely pruritic plaques; Sézary cells seen on peripheral blood smear; treat with chemotherapy.

◘ **Erythroderma** A systemic skin inflammation that is either idiopathic or secondary to underlying dermatologic disease (e.g., psoriasis, dermatitis), cutaneous lymphomas, or drug reactions; presents with generalized pruritic erythema with lichenification and secondary scaling; may desquamate; treat with corticosteroids and moisturizers; treat the underlying condition if it can be determined; complications include secondary infections, folate deficiency

◘ **Hairy Cell Leukemia** Chronic B-cell leukemia seen primarily in men > 40 years of age; presents with weakness, gingival bleeding, abdominal mass, recurrent bacterial infections, and splenomegaly; anemia and pancytopenia; hairy cells (B-cells with thin, long cytoplasmic projections) seen; treat with purine analogs (cladribine), pentostatin, or alpha-interferon; consider splenectomy; with treatment, prognosis is much better than that of other chronic leukemias.

◘ **Waldenström's Macroglobulinemia** A B-lymphocyte disorder with excessive IgM production and hyperviscosity syndrome; presents with visual disturbances, easy bruising, bleeding gums, engorgement of the retinal veins, lymphadenopathy, and hepatosplenomegaly; rouleaux formation, monoclonal IgM spike on serum electrophoresis, and increased serum viscosity; bone marrow is characteristically infiltrated by plasmacytic lymphocytes; treat with plasmapheresis, chlorambucil, cyclophosphamide.

ID/CC	A **46-year-old male** complains of **easy fatigability** and **weakness**.
HPI	He acknowledges recent **weight loss, anorexia, abdominal fullness** (due to massive splenomegaly), and **night sweats**.
PE	VS: **low-grade fever** (38.5 C). PE: pallor; no lymphadenopathy; **splenomegaly** palpable 10 cm below costal margin; hepatomegaly.
Labs	CBC/PBS: **elevated WBC** (> 100,000); decreased hemoglobin (9); thrombocytosis; **many mature neutrophils, promyelocytes, metamyelocytes, and myelocytes** (< 10% myeloblasts). Serum B_{12} and uric acid elevated; decreased leukocyte alkaline phosphatase; **bone marrow biopsy reveals hypercellularity with elevated myeloid–erythroid ratio** (10:1); **translocation** (9:22) (q34; q11) (= BCR-ABL FUSION GENE OR PHILADELPHIA CHROMOSOME).
Imaging	N/A.
Pathogenesis	Chronic myelogenous leukemia (CML) is a **myeloproliferative disease** that is characterized by clonal expansion of neoplastic pluripotent stem cells. In > 90% of cases, the disease arises following the formation of the **bcr-abl fusion gene,** which produces an abnormal tyrosine kinase.
Epidemiology	Occurs most commonly in the fourth to fifth decades with a **slight male predominance** and accounts for 15%–20% of all leukemia cases. Survivors of the atomic bomb in Japan developed CML at an increased, dose-dependent rate, with most cases arising 5–12 years after exposure. Median survival is approximately 3–4 years.
Management	For patients who can tolerate transplant and who have donors, **allogenic bone marrow transplant** often offers the best hope for cure. Others are offered **alpha-interferon,** which may induce remission in some patients. Patients in the chronic phase are frequently given **hydroxyurea** to minimize the leukemic cell burden. CML has a **biphasic** or **triphasic** clinical course. The **chronic phase** behaves as a benign neoplasm and can be managed with chemotherapy or immunotherapy. CML progresses to a **blastic phase** that resembles acute

leukemia with or without an intervening **accelerated phase.**

Complications Hyperviscosity and/or thrombocytosis; predisposition to cerebrovascular accidents, neuropathies, and splenic infarcts.

Associated Diseases ◘ **Essential Thrombocytosis** Idiopathic overproduction of platelets; presents with markedly increased platelet counts (typically > 1 million); patients may have ecchymoses due to ineffective platelets; treat with hydroxyurea; follow with repeated CBCs and marrow biopsies, as the disease can progress to myelofibrosis or leukemia.

◘ **Polycythemia Vera** Idiopathic proliferation of erythroid stem cells; presents with epistaxis, melena, DVT, pruritus, plethora, and splenomegaly; markedly increased RBC count, variably elevated WBCs and platelets, normal arterial PO_2, and low erythropoietin levels (to distinguish from secondary polycythemia); treat with phlebotomy, hydroxyurea; complications include CNS artery thrombosis and progression to leukemia.

ID/CC	A 42-year-old woman hospitalized in the ICU for *E. coli* **sepsis** begins to display extensive skin and mucous membrane **bleeding.**
HPI	She is being treated with IV antibiotics and is on pressor therapy.
PE	VS: tachycardia (HR 129); hypotension (BP 66/42); breathing with assisted ventilation. PE: unresponsive; multiple **diffuse petechiae** and **hematomas;** bleeding from IV and pulmonary artery catheter sites.
Labs	CBC: thrombocytopenia. PBS: schistocytes. Prolonged PT/PTT; low fibrinogen; low clotting factors; elevated fibrin degradation products; elevated D dimer.
Imaging	N/A
Pathogenesis	Disseminated intravascular coagulation (DIC) is characterized by a generalized activation of the coagulation system that may present with varying degrees of severity. It is most frequently associated with obstetrical complications (amniotic fluid embolism, intrauterine fetal death, septic abortion), metastatic malignancy, massive trauma, and bacterial sepsis. Pathophysiologically, a potent thrombogenic stimulus causes thrombosis production throughout the microvasculature followed by a hemorrhagic phase marked by procoagulant factor consumption and secondary fibrinolysis.
Epidemiology	N/A
Management	**Correct the underlying disorder** (e.g., infection). Control bleeding or thrombosis. Administer fresh frozen plasma to replace depleted clotting factors, blood and platelet concentrates to correct thrombocytopenia, and low-dose **IV heparin** in cases of thrombosis. Treat chronic DIC with periodic plasma and platelet replacement. DIC is unresponsive to warfarin; heparin may be administered by periodic injection or continuous infusion.
Complications	Complications include uncontrollable hemorrhage, ARDS, thrombosis of vessels, and pregangrenous changes in the digits, nose, and genitalia.

....

47. **DISSEMINATED INTRAVASCULAR COAGULATION**

Microinfarctions and thrombi can also be found in the heart, liver, kidneys, and brain.

◻ **Hemolytic-Uremic Syndrome** Acute renal failure and microangiopathic hemolytic anemia, usually associated with bacterial (*E. coli*, *Shigella*) infection in children or following cancer chemotherapy (mitomycin); presents with fever, malaise, hypotension, ecchymoses, periorbital edema, and oliguria; schistocytes seen on PBS; no evidence of DIC (normal PT, PTT, fibrinogen); thrombocytopenia and elevated BUN and creatinine; treat with plasmapheresis, IV fluids and pressors as needed to prevent acute renal failure and hemodynamic compromise.

◻ **Heparin Toxicity** Acute hemorrhage due to overdosing or to autoimmune thrombocytopenia as a side effect of appropriate dosing; presents with extensive ecchymoses and hemorrhage; thrombocytopenia, markedly prolonged PTT in overdosage; treat with discontinuation of heparin, protamine sulfate, blood and platelet transfusions as needed.

◻ **Thrombotic Thrombocytopenic Purpura** An idiopathic disease found in pregnant and HIV-positive patients and after exposure to antibiotics or estrogens; presents with episodic altered mental status, fever, renal dysfunction, petechiae over the chest and extremities, and fever; anemia, schistocytes on smear, low platelet count, and absent haptoglobin; treat with plasmapheresis.

◻ **Sepsis** A systemic inflammatory condition due to overwhelming infection; presents with diaphoresis, clammy skin, tachypnea, hypotension, and fever or hypothermia; leukocytosis with left shift; blood and urine cultures may be positive; treat with IV antibiotics, fluids and pressors as needed.

DISSEMINATED INTRAVASCULAR COAGULATION

ID/CC	A 29-year-old male presents complaining of **easy fatigability and lethargy.**
HPI	The patient states that he was diagnosed with **gallstones** several years ago and adds that his **mother had a splenectomy** while in her 20s.
PE	VS: normal. PE: **jaundice; scleral icterus;** abdomen soft, nontender, and nondistended; **splenomegaly.**
Labs	CBC: normal WBC; **decreased hemoglobin (9.5) and hematocrit (28); slightly decreased MCV; elevated MCHC. [A]** PBS: anisocytosis with numerous spherocytes; reticulocytosis. LFTs: unconjugated bilirubin elevated. Osmotic fragility test positive.
Imaging	N/A
Pathogenesis	Hereditary spherocytosis (HS) is an **autosomal-dominant** disorder characterized by cytoskeletal defects in the RBC membrane, yielding RBCs that are spheroidal, more rigid, fragile, and at risk for splenic sequestration and lysis. The **most common defect occurs in spectrin,** a cytoskeletal element that ordinarily acts as a strut to support the RBC membrane and maintain its biconcave disk shape. Infection, particularly with parvovirus B19, may precipitate decompensation and aplastic crisis.
Epidemiology	HS occasionally appears in infancy but is often clinically inapparent until adulthood.
Management	RBC survival is dramatically enhanced with **splenectomy** despite the persistence of the cytoskeletal abnormality. Do not schedule splenectomy until after four years of age because of the risk of severe infection. Administer **polyvalent pneumococcal vaccine** prior to surgery. Give folic acid and iron supplementation as needed.
Complications	Chronic leg ulcers, gallstones, and folate deficiency. **FIRST AID 2** p. 164
Associated Diseases	N/A

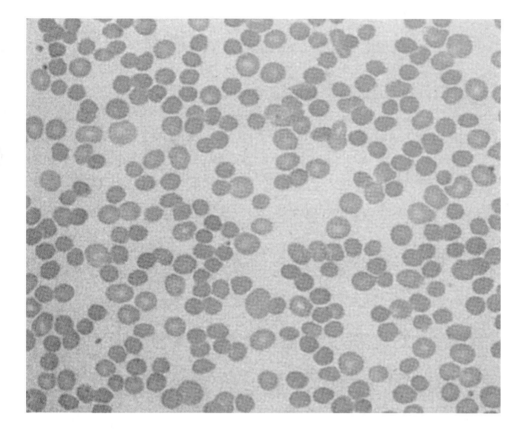

HEREDITARY SPHEROCYTOSIS

ID/CC	A **35-year-old man** has been troubled by **fever, weight loss,** and drenching **night sweats** for the past several weeks.
HPI	He has no significant medical history.
PE	VS: fever (38.9 C). PE: **[A]** nontender cervical lymphadenopathy; hepatosplenomegaly.
Labs	CBC: anemia; leukocytosis. Elevated ESR. LFTs: elevated serum alkaline phosphatase; elevated LDH. **[B]** lymph node biopsy reveals **binucleate giant cell** with eosinophilic inclusion-like nucleoli (= REED–STERNBERG CELL).
Imaging	**[C]** CXR-PA: widespread enlargement of hilar and mediastinal lymph nodes.
Pathogenesis	The etiology is unknown, although all forms are characterized by the presence of the Reed–Sternberg (RS) cell, a large cell with bilobate nucleoli. Hodgkin's lymphoma is categorized in four forms: (1) **lymphocytic predominance,** which is the least common form, carries the best prognosis, and is characterized by a predominance of lymphocytic cells compared to RS cells; (2) **mixed cellularity,** which is associated with a good prognosis; (3) **lymphocytic depletion,** which carries the worst prognosis and is characterized by a proliferation of RS cells and a depletion of lymphocytes; and (4) **nodular sclerosis,** which is the most common form, carries a good prognosis, and is characterized by nodular division of affected lymph nodes by fibrous bands and by the presence of lacunar cells.
Epidemiology	The incidence of Hodgkin's lymphoma is **higher in men** (commonly occurring between 15 and 35 years of age, with another peak in those > 50 years) than in women except for the nodular sclerosis form.
Management	**Radiation** is indicated for focal disease (stage IA or IIA). Disseminated disease should be treated with aggressive **combination chemotherapy.** The treatment of choice appears to be doxorubicin, bleomycin, vincristine, and dacarbazine. A combination of therapies may be indicated for advanced disease.
Complications	Chemotherapeutic modalities used (MOPP, ABVD) may be associated with a long-term risk of secondary

HODGKIN'S LYMPHOMA

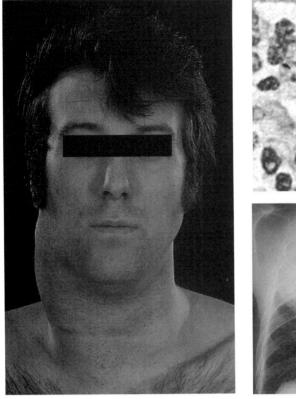

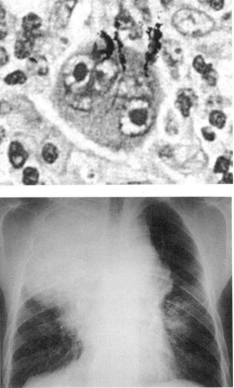

leukemias and infertility. Mediastinal irradiation leads to paresthesias, sclerosis of coronary arteries (increased risk of MI), pulmonary fibrosis, pericardial effusions, and hypothyroidism.

Associated Diseases

■ **Non-Hodgkin's Lymphoma** A lymphoid tissue malignancy occurring anywhere in the body; presents with firm lymphadenopathy, fever, night sweats, and weight loss; anemia and elevated LDH; lymph nodes with "cut potato" appearance; treat with combination chemotherapy, surgery and radiotherapy if localized.

ID/CC	A 29-year-old **female** presents to the clinic complaining of **persistent fatigue and weakness.**
HPI	She states that she has **heavy menstrual bleeding** (= MENORRHAGIA) and frequent **bleeding between periods** (= METRORRHAGIA). She adds that she has **brittle nails** and frequently **eats ice** (= PAGOPHAGIA).
PE	VS: normal. PE: **pallor;** no scleral icterus; moist mucous membranes; **atrophic tongue;** 2-sec capillary refill; regular rate and rhythm.
Labs	CBC/PBS: **[A]** **hypochromic, microcytic RBCs; low hemoglobin (9) and hematocrit (28); elevated RDW; low MCV and MCHC.** Serum iron depressed; ferritin low; TIBC elevated.
Imaging	N/A
Pathogenesis	Iron is absorbed preferentially in the duodenum and proximal jejunum, so conditions that bypass or otherwise decrease absorption may lead to anemia. Iron deficiency may also develop in conditions where blood is lost through the **GI** (peptic ulcer, gastritis, hemorrhoids, angiodysplasia, parasites, and malignancy) **or GU tract, in menstruation,** and in conditions of **increased iron demand such as pregnancy or adolescence.** Depleted iron stores result in hemoglobin-deficient cells and consequent hypochromia and microcytosis.
Epidemiology	Iron deficiency is the **most common form of anemia** in the U.S., appearing in **20% of U.S. women.**
Management	Oral ferrous sulfate will yield a brisk reticulocytosis within 3–4 days and a substantial increase in hemoglobin in approximately 10 days. In patients who are unable to tolerate oral ferrous sulfate, oral ferrous gluconate and fumarate as well as a parenteral formulation are available.
Complications	Complications include high-output cardiac failure and Plummer–Vinson syndrome. **FIRST AID 2** p. 163
Associated Diseases	◘ **Lead Toxicity** Ingestion of gasoline, wall paint, or clay utensils; presents with acute or subacute altered mental status, mental retardation in children, peripheral neuropathy, colicky abdominal pain, fatigue, ataxia, and purple lead lines on gums; microcytic anemia with basophilic stippling, elevated blood lead levels, and

IRON DEFICIENCY ANEMIA

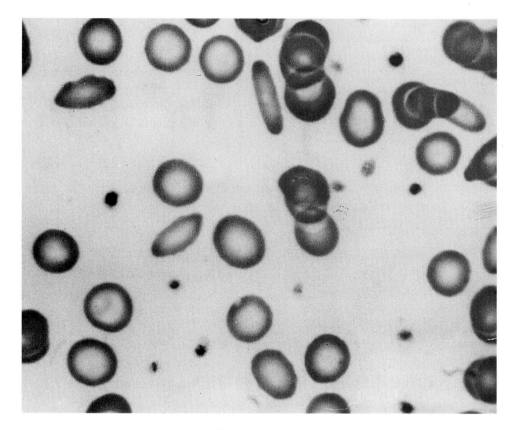

elevated free erythrocyte protoporphyrin; XR shows broad bands of increased density in long bones; treat with EDTA, dimercaprol chelation, and avoidance of exposure.

◻ **Paroxysmal Nocturnal Hemoglobinuria** An acquired RBC membrane defect (absence of decay-accelerating factor, or DAF); erythrocytes are unusually sensitive to complement-mediated destruction; presents with nocturnal intravascular hemolysis (abdominal and lumbar pain, brown urine, pallor) and increased tendency toward venous thrombosis (may result in Budd–Chiari syndrome, sagittal sinus thrombosis, etc.); anemia, hemoglobinemia and hemoglobinuria, decreased haptoglobin, and elevated LDH; acidified serum hemolysis test positive; absence of DAF (most sensitive and specific test) on RBCs demonstrated by flow cytometry; treat acutely with corticosteroids, transfuse as needed.

◻ **Plummer–Vinson Syndrome** Iron deficiency; common in young females; presents with dysphagia, pica, koilonychia, and glossitis; microcytic anemia; UGI shows esophageal webbing; treat with esophageal dilatation, iron supplementation; complications include a predisposition to esophageal carcinoma.

ID/CC	A **59-year-old black male** seeks attention for **lower back pain.**
HPI	He also complains of **fatigue** and **rib tenderness.**
PE	VS: normal. PE: **pallor;** petechiae on buccal mucosa; **bone tenderness** on pressing ribs and spine; no hepatosplenomegaly; blanching and cyanosis of fingers, toes, tips of nose, and earlobes (= RAYNAUD'S PHENOMENON).
Labs	CBC/PBS: normocytic **anemia** (Hb 8.0); **leukopenia;** [A] rouleaux formation. **Markedly elevated ESR. Hypercalcemia; hypogammaglobulinemia;** increased serum total protein; serum protein electrophoresis shows a **monoclonal spike** (M protein) on beta or gamma globulin region (= MONOCLONAL GAMMOPATHY); [B] bone marrow shows replacement of normal marrow elements by plasma cells. UA: increased uric acid; phosphaturia; glucosuria; **Bence Jones proteinuria** (IgG light chains).
Imaging	[C] XR-Skull: punched-out (= OSTEOLYTIC) lesions in the skull with generalized **osteoporosis** (bone scan is not useful; no uptake due to lack of osteoblastic component).
Pathogenesis	A primary malignant neoplastic proliferation of plasma cells in the bone marrow with resulting marrow failure and overproduction of immunoglobulin. Serum immunoelectrophoresis shows a monoclonal elevation of one immunoglobulin (detected by serum protein electrophoresis) with a reciprocal depression of the other classes of immunoglobulins. The bone pain and lesions result from tumor growth and from increased osteoclast activity (induced by cytokines produced by myeloma cells). Pneumonia and UTIs are common because of the abnormal immunoglobulin profile. Renal failure (25% of patients) results from several contributing factors, including hypercalcemia, infection, and the excretion of light chains.
Epidemiology	**The most common primary bone tumor** in adults. Median age at presentation is 60; mean survival after diagnosis (without treatment) is 30 months. More common in blacks.
Management	Administer **systemic chemotherapy** (alkylating agents

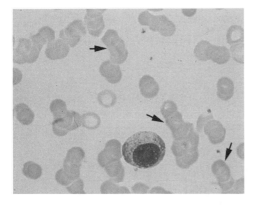 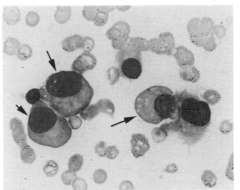

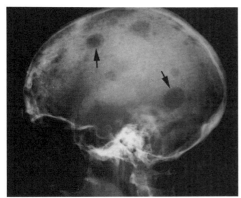

are used most commonly); bone lesions require **biphosphonates** and **local radiation** to prevent pathologic fracture. Give **IV gamma globulin** to correct profound hypogammaglobulinemia and reduce infections; **treat hypercalcemia;** manage pain; **bone marrow transplant** in refractory cases. Administer **pneumococcal vaccine.**

Complications

Hyperviscosity syndrome (visual and mental status disturbances, vertigo, headache, and mucosal bleeding), cryoglobulinemia, pathologic fractures (possibly leading to spinal cord compression, carpal tunnel syndrome, etc.), recurrent infections, sepsis, **amyloidosis, light chain nephropathy** with renal failure, and peripheral neuropathy (due to amyloidosis).

Associated Diseases

☐ **Amyloidosis** Systemic deposition of one of several types of proteins within multiple organs; can be idiopathic; associated with diseases such as multiple myeloma or secondary to chronic inflammatory processes; presents with dysfunction of multiple organs, including nephrotic syndrome, cardiomyopathy, hepatomegaly, and hypothyroidism; biopsy demonstrates apple-green birefringence after Congo red staining of tissues; treat the underlying cause (e.g., myeloma); consider organ transplant.

◻ **Monoclonal Gammopathy of Undetermined Significance** Overproduction of antibody by a single B-cell clone; incidence increases with advancing age; typically asymptomatic; immunoelectrophoresis shows spike of homogenous immunoglobulin; treatment is not required, but patients should be closely followed, as approximately 33% with MGUS go on to develop diseases such as multiple myeloma, amyloidosis, and lymphoid malignancies.

ID/CC	A 61-year-old male complains of **painless lumps** (= LYMPHADENOPATHY) in his neck and groin that have been increasing in size.
HPI	He additionally reports **mild fever, weight loss,** and **night sweats** over the past three months.
PE	VS: low-grade fever (38.3 C). PE: pallor; cervical, axillary, and femoral lymphadenopathy; large mass in **Waldeyer's ring; splenomegaly.**
Labs	CBC: Coombs-positive hemolytic **anemia;** thrombocytopenia. Elevated serum LDH; hypergammaglobulinemia. LP: no malignant cells in CSF. **[A]** Lymph node dissection reveals lymphoid follicles throughout lymph node. **[B]** In another type of non-Hodgkin's lymphoma, lymph nodes are diffusely infiltrated by lymphoma cells.
Imaging	CXR/CT-Chest, Pelvis, Abdomen: lymphadenopathy and organ involvement; assess the spread of disease.
Pathogenesis	Non-Hodgkin's lymphomas are malignant neoplasms arising from lymphoid cells or other cells native to lymphoid tissue. They are classified on the basis of histopathologic cell type (small lymphocytic, follicular, cleaved large cell, histiocytic, lymphoblastic, etc.). Staging of the disease is as follows: **stage I:** involvement of a single lymph node region or extralymphatic site. **Stage II:** involvement of two or more lymph node areas on the same side of the diaphragm. **Stage III:** involvement of lymph node areas on both sides of the diaphragm (many include spleen). **Stage IV:** one or more extralymphatic organs (with or without lymphatic spread).
Epidemiology	Small cell lymphocytic, follicular small cell cleaved, and large cell immunoblastic are most common in older adults, although the immunoblastic form may also be found in children. Individuals with HIV are particularly prone to immunoblastic lymphoma of the CNS. Lymphoblastic and small cell uncleaved lymphomas are most common in children.
Management	Staging (e.g., bone or gallium scan, LP) and tumor histology direct treatment. Aggressive **combination chemotherapy** is the mainstay of treatment for high-

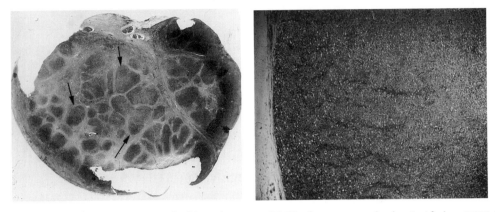

grade lymphomas CNS chemoprophylaxis if the CSF is free of tumor. Surgery or radiation therapy for large obstructive or bulky tumors; prophylaxis for prevention of tumor lysis syndrome with allopurinol, aggressive IV volume expansion, and alkalinization of urine (increases uric acid excretion). In general, patients with low-grade disease survive long but are rarely cured; high-grade tumors respond well to treatment and may be cured.

Complications Complications include superior vena cava syndrome, metastasis, and bowel obstruction. Tumor lysis syndrome may cause hyperkalemia, hypocalcemia, hyperphosphatemia, and hyperuricemia. Common chemotherapeutic complications include bone marrow suppression, hemorrhagic cystitis (cyclophosphamide), cardiomyopathy (doxorubicin/adriamycin), pulmonary fibrosis (bleomycin), peripheral neuropathy and weakness (vincristine), and hypertension (prednisone).

Associated Diseases ❑ **Hodgkin's Lymphoma** Malignancy of lymphoid tissue, linked in some patients to EBV infection; presents with generalized lymphadenopathy, hepatosplenomegaly, fever, night sweats, and weight loss, or may present with asymptomatic adenopathy; chest and abdominal CT may reveal adenopathy and hepatosplenomegaly; lymph node biopsy shows Reed–Sternberg cells (necessary but not sufficient for diagnosis); treat with radiation therapy for local disease, allowing a nearly 90% five-year survival rate; add chemotherapy for metastatic disease.

ID/CC	A **62-year-old** white **male** complains of increasing **headaches, dizziness,** and **fatigue** over the past month.
HPI	The patient reports that his headaches have become more frequent and have been accompanied by **ringing in the ears** (= TINNITUS) and **blurry vision.** The patient additionally notes **generalized itching** following warm showers (due to histamine release).
PE	VS: hypertension. PE: **facial plethora; engorged retinal veins;** neurologic exam nonfocal; **mild hepatomegaly; splenomegaly.**
Labs	CBC: **hematocrit elevated** (> 60); **elevated RBC mass; elevated WBC count** (13,000); **thrombocytosis** (600,000). PBS: **normal RBC morphology.** ABGs: normal. **Low erythropoietin;** elevated vitamin B_{12} levels (due to increased transcobalamin III levels); elevated leukocyte alkaline phosphatase; elevated uric acid.
Imaging	N/A
Pathogenesis	An acquired **myeloproliferative disorder** that is characterized by overproduction of all three hematopoietic cell lines with predominant elevation in RBCs. This overproduction is **independent of erythropoietin.**
Epidemiology	Relatively common; seen more frequently in **males** (60%) and presents most commonly in late middle life (**median age 60** at presentation). The disease is uncommon among blacks.
Management	Periodic **phlebotomy** to reduce the hematocrit to < 46%. Iron deficiency is inevitable in many patients with continued phlebotomy; iron supplementation may be required. **Myelosuppressive therapy** may be indicated if patients develop a high phlebotomy requirement, thrombocytosis, or intractable pruritus. **Hydroxyurea** achieves long-term disease control in most patients. Alkylating agents should be avoided because of leukemogenic potential. **Alpha-interferon** may be used in combination with intermittent phlebotomy or hydroxyurea in refractory patients. A reduction of platelet count to < 700,000 reduces the risk of thrombotic complications; thus, patients may benefit from antiplatelet agents and/or anticoagulants.

POLYCYTHEMIA VERA

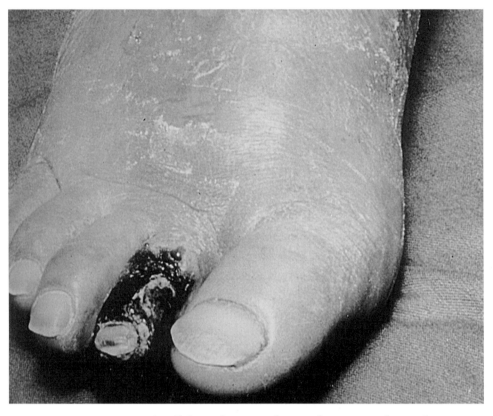

Antihistamines can be used to control pruritus.

Complications Polycythemia vera has a median survival of 6–8 months untreated and 11–12 years with adequate therapy. Most complications, such as **[A]** gangrene, are attributable to vascular thrombosis (hyperviscosity). Hemorrhage can result from peptic ulcer formation (dysfunctional platelets, increased histamine and gastric acid production); hyperuricemia may result from increased cell turnover. Patients who reach the "spent" or "burnt-out" phase develop marked splenomegaly and anemia associated with bone marrow fibrosis. Such patients may experience conversion to myelofibrosis or chronic myelogenous leukemia. Acute myelogenous leukemia may also develop in 2%–5% of patients. Hyperviscosity syndrome may also occur as a result of the elevated hematocrit.

Associated Diseases ◘ **Essential Thrombocytosis** Idiopathic overproduction of platelets; presents with markedly increased platelet counts (typically > 1 million); patients may have ecchymoses due to ineffective platelets; treat with hydroxyurea; follow with repeated CBCs and marrow biopsies, as the disease can progress to myelofibrosis or leukemia.

ID/CC	A 33-year-old **Chinese** woman is found to have a low hematocrit on routine screening labs.
HPI	The patient is otherwise healthy with no complaints. She recalls having had a previous bout with anemia during childhood but denies any hemoptysis, hematochezia, melena, menorrhagia, gross hematuria, or other bleeding tendencies. Her **brother had a similar anemia** in childhood and has always had "low blood."
PE	VS: normal. PE: conjunctiva pale; no petechiae or ecchymoses noted; lung, cardiac, and abdominal exams normal; rectal exam normal with heme-negative stool.
Labs	CBC/PBS: **low hemoglobin** (9.4) **and hematocrit** (28.9); **[A]** microcytes; hypochromia; occasional target cells (1); **low MCV** (69). **Iron studies normal;** normal reticulocyte count; hemoglobin electrophoresis reveals **normal HgA and HgA2.**
Imaging	N/A
Pathogenesis	Thalassemia is a hereditary disorder that results from impaired production of globin chains (alpha or beta) that leads to a defective hemoglobin structure within RBCs and to a hypochromic, microcytic anemia. **Alpha-thalassemias** are due to **gene deletions** that directly cause reduced alpha-globin chain synthesis with no effect on HgA, HgA2, or HgF structure. Excess beta chains in the severe form may produce a B4 tetramer (HgH). **Beta-thalassemias** are usually caused by **point mutations** that result in reduced or absent beta-globin synthesis, which is classified as either no synthesis (B0) or reduced synthesis (B+). Excess alpha chains that are produced are unstable and can precipitate, thus damaging RBC membranes and causing intramedullary hemolysis and resultant bone marrow hyperplasia. Homozygous disease (thalassemia major) presents as severe transfusion-requiring anemia during the first year of life, usually occurring after six months, when hemoglobin synthesis shifts from HgF to HgA.
Epidemiology	**Alpha-thalassemias** are seen in individuals from Southeast Asia or China and, less commonly, in blacks. **Beta-thalassemia** usually affects individuals of Mediterranean origin (Greek or Italian) and, less

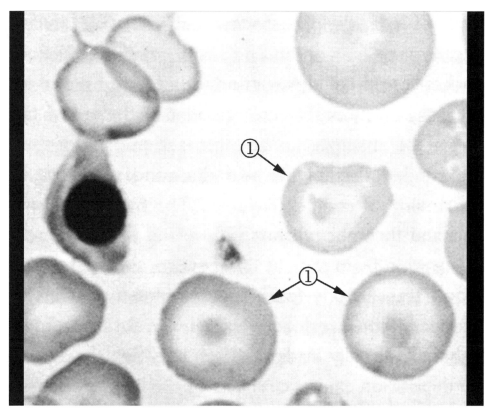

commonly, Chinese, Asians, and blacks.

Management This patient has asymptomatic alpha-thalassemia, for which no treatment is indicated. **Regular transfusions** and **folate supplementation** are indicated for severe beta-thalassemia (= COOLEY'S ANEMIA). Patients with the HgH variant require transfusions only during acute hemolytic exacerbations. **Splenectomy** is performed when hypersplenism increases the requirement for more frequent transfusions. **Deferoxamine** is routinely offered as an iron-chelating agent to prevent or postpone hemosiderosis. **Allogeneic bone marrow transplantation** is now an option for beta-thalassemic children who have yet to develop iron overload or chronic organ toxicity.

Complications Untreated chronic iron overload secondary to thalassemia may result in **cardiomyopathy,** progressive hepatomegaly, and endocrine dysfunction. Death from **cardiac failure** may occur by the third decade.

Associated Diseases ☐ **Anemia of Chronic Disease** Anemia due to unspecified inflammatory mediators released during chronic diseases (e.g., arthritis, malignancy, or infection); presents with fatigue, weakness, tachycardia, and flow murmur; microcytic, hypochromic anemia with low serum iron and low serum TIBC; ferritin is often elevated; treat underlying disease.

◘ **Lead Toxicity** Ingestion of gasoline, wall paint, or clay utensils; presents with acute or subacute altered mental status, mental retardation in children, peripheral neuropathy, colicky abdominal pain, fatigue, ataxia, and purple lead lines on gums; microcytic anemia with basophilic stippling, elevated blood lead levels, and elevated free erythrocyte protoporphyrin; XR shows broad bands of increased density in long bones; treat with EDTA, dimercaprol chelation, and avoidance of exposure.

◘ **Sideroblastic Anemia** Hypochromic anemia, congenital or acquired, associated with an abnormal erythroid precursor, "ringed sideroblast," leading to defects in the porphyrin pathway; presents with weakness, fatigue, and pallor; elevated serum iron and increased transferrin saturation; ringed sideroblasts seen with special stain of red cells; treat with pyridoxine supplements, blood cell transfusions; consider deferoxamine iron chelation.

ID/CC	A **28-year-old female** is brought to the emergency room after having a **seizure** at work.
HPI	The patient has experienced similar episodes in the past and also complains of increased **fatigue.** She first noticed these symptoms several weeks ago but has only recently sought care.
PE	VS: tachycardia (HR 126); **fever** (39.3 C). PE: multiple **petechiae;** no hepatosplenomegaly; neurologic examination normal.
Labs	CBC/PBS: **thrombocytopenia** (53,000); **elevated reticulocyte count; schistocytes;** helmet cells; **altered platelet morphology.** LDH increased; PT/PTT normal; fibrinogen concentrations normal. UA: proteinuria.
Imaging	N/A
Pathogenesis	Thrombotic thrombocytopenic purpura (TTP) is characterized by the presence of **microangiopathic hemolytic anemia, thrombocytopenia, neurologic disorders, renal dysfunction**, and **fever.** Its precise etiology is unknown, but a strong immunologic component is suspected. Pathologically, localized arteriolar thrombi and fibrin deposition produce most disease manifestations.
Epidemiology	TTP affects people of all ages but primarily **young women.**
Management	**Glucocorticoids,** splenectomy, and antiplatelet drugs are used with some success. Antiplatelet drugs (aspirin, dextran, dipyridamole, and sulfinpyrazone) may be used in conjunction with other treatments. Acute life-threatening complications require emergent exchange transfusion or plasmapheresis coupled with infusion of fresh frozen plasma. Patients are at risk of death or coma. Remission occurs in two-thirds of patients if treated promptly.
Complications	Patients may develop GI or GU hemorrhage, pancreatitis, progressive CNS dysfunction (delirium, confusion, seizure, aphasia, and visual field deficits), or renal failure. May be fatal. Relapses occur in 10% of cases.

....

55. **THROMBOTIC THROMBOCYTOPENIC PURPURA**

◻ **Hemolytic-Uremic Syndrome** Acute renal failure and microangiopathic hemolytic anemia, usually associated with bacterial (*E. coli, Shigella*) infection in children or following cancer chemotherapy (mitomycin); presents with fever, malaise, hypotension, ecchymoses, periorbital edema, and oliguria; schistocytes seen on PBS; no evidence of DIC (normal PT, PTT, fibrinogen); thrombocytopenia and elevated BUN and creatinine; treat with plasmapheresis, IV fluids and pressors as needed to prevent acute renal failure and hemodynamic compromise.

◻ **Idiopathic Thrombocytopenic Purpura** Autoantibodies against platelets; affects children and young adults; often preceded by viral illness; presents with epistaxis and purpura; no palpable spleen; isolated thrombocytopenia and normal bone marrow with increased megakaryocytes; treat with high-dose prednisone, splenectomy.

THROMBOTIC THROMBOCYTOPENIC PURPURA

ID/CC	A 50-year-old **vegan** woman presents with **pallor** and **fatigue**.
HPI	She also reports **spastic weakness** of both legs and **anesthesia** progressing proximally from her distal extremities (= GLOVE-AND-STOCKING DISTRIBUTION).
PE	VS: normal. PE: pallor; mild icterus; **beefy-red tongue** (= GLOSSITIS); **loss of balance, vibratory, and position sense** in both lower extremities; decreased sensation in distal extremities; spastic weakness of lower extremities with absent DTRs; Babinski's present bilaterally; hepatosplenomegaly.
Labs	CBC / PBS: **decreased hemoglobin; high MCV** (= MACROCYTIC ANEMIA); mild leukopenia (4,000) with [A] **hypersegmented neutrophils;** thrombocytopenia. Low serum cobalamin; achlorhydria (no hydrochloric acid in gastric juice); Schilling test consistent with **intrinsic factor deficiency**; antibodies against parietal cells and intrinsic factor demonstrated; homocysteinemia; hypomethioninemia. UA: homocysteinuria.
Imaging	N/A
Pathogenesis	The absorption of vitamin B_{12} (also known as cobalamin) requires (1) adequate dietary intake (vitamin B_{12} is found only in animal products); (2) production of intrinsic factor by the gastric antrum; and (3) uptake of the intrinsic factor–vitamin complex by the terminal ileum. Deficiency of vitamin B_{12} may have various causes; atrophic gastritis results in decreased intrinsic factor production with subsequent malabsorption of vitamin B_{12}. The same effect results from antral resection. Diseases affecting the terminal ileum (e.g., Crohn's disease and intestinal lymphoma) can prevent the uptake of the intrinsic factor–vitamin B_{12} complex. Blind-loop syndrome results in bacterial overgrowth within the intestine, resulting in consumption of vitamin B_{12} before uptake can occur. In severe cases of malnutrition (e.g., alcoholism), vitamin B_{12} deficiency may occur because of decreased intake. The Schilling test is designed to identify the cause of vitamin B_{12} deficiency.
Epidemiology	More common among patients with chronic malnutrition and among those with minimal or no meat

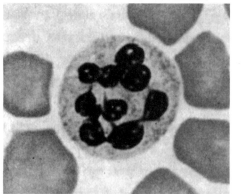
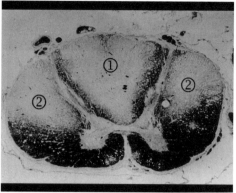

consumption (vegetarians).

Management **Lifelong, regular IM vitamin B$_{12}$ supplementation.**

Complications Macrocytic, megaloblastic anemia, glossitis, confusion, depression, psychosis ("megaloblastic madness"), decreased phagocyte and PMN response, **[B]** subacute combined degeneration of the spinal cord with characteristic involvement of posterior (1) and lateral (2) tracts, and progressive peripheral neuropathy.

Associated Diseases ◘ **Folate Deficiency** Folate is required for DNA/RNA synthesis; deficiency is most commonly associated with alcoholism, pregnancy, or medications (Bactrim, methotrexate, phenytoin); presents with fatigue, weakness, and nausea; anemia, hypersegmented PMNs, megaloblastic RBCs, and low RBC folate; treat with folic acid supplementation; folic acid is required for patients taking Bactrim or methotrexate.

◘ **Pernicious Anemia** An autoimmune disorder most often seen in the elderly; causes vitamin B$_{12}$ deficiency due to decreased intrinsic factor (IF) activity; presents with pallor, fatigue, chronic atrophic gastritis, subacute combined degeneration of the spinal cord (especially the posterior columns and the corticospinal tracts), peripheral neuropathy, and cognitive deficits; megaloblastic anemia and hypersegmented neutrophils; Schilling test positive; reduced vitamin B$_{12}$ levels and anti-IF and anti-parietal cell antibodies; treat with lifelong intramuscular vitamin B$_{12}$; complications include increased risk of gastric carcinoma with chronic atrophic gastritis.

From the authors of *Underground Clinical Vignettes*

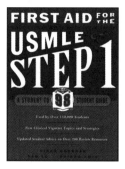

A true classic used by over 200,000 students around the world. The '99 edition features details on the new computerized test, new color plates and thoroughly updated high-yield facts and book reviews. Bi-directional links with the *Underground Clinical Vignettes Step 1* series. ISBN 0-8385-2612-8.

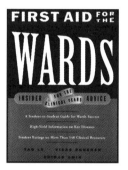

This high-yield student-to-student guide is designed to help students make the transition from the basic sciences to the hospital wards and succeed on their clinical rotations. The book features an orientation to the hospital environment, tips on being an effective and efficient junior medical student, student-proven advice tailored to each core rotation, a database of high-yield clinical facts, and recommendations for clinical pocket books, texts, and references. ISBN 0-8385-2595-4.

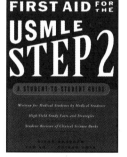

This entirely rewritten second edition now follows in the footsteps of *First Aid for the USMLE Step 1*. Features an exam preparation guide geared to the new computerized test, basic science and clinical high-yield facts, color plates and ratings of USMLE Step 2 books and software. Bi-directional links with the *Underground Clinical Vignettes Step 2* series.

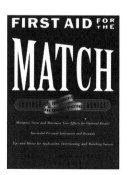

This top rated (5 stars, *Doody Review*) student-to-student guide helps medical students effectively and efficiently navigate the residency application process, helping them make the most of their limited time, money, and energy. The book draws on the advice and experiences of successful student applicants as well as residency directors. Also featured are application and interview tips tailored to each specialty, successful personal statements and CVs with analyses, current trends, and common interview questions with suggested strategies for responding. ISBN 0-8385-2596-2.

The *First Aid* series by Appleton & Lange...the review book leader.
Available through your local health sciences bookstore !